Julia's Story

Other Books by Fred J. Cook

The Unfinished Story of Alger Hiss
What Manner of Men
A Two-Dollar Bet Means Murder
The Warfare State
The F.B.I. Nobody Knows
The Corrupted Land
The Secret Rulers
The Plot Against the Patient
What So Proudly We Hailed
The Nightmare Decade

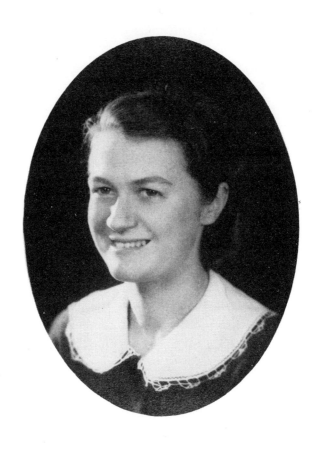

FRED J. COOK

Julia's Story

The Tragedy of an Unnecessary Death

HOLT, RINEHART AND WINSTON
New York

Library of Congress Cataloging in Publication Data

Cook, Fred J
    Julia's story.

    1. Heart—Surgery—Personal narratives. 2. Cook,
Julia. 3. Postoperative care. 4. Hospital care—
United States. I. Title.
RD598.C65   362.1'9'612700924 [B]   75-21626
ISBN 0-03-014726-3

Printed in the United States of America

Part of this book first appeared in slightly different form in
New York magazine.

10 9 8 7 6 5 4 3 2 1

To the Memory of the Girl
I Will Never Forget

Julia's Story

1

OUR NERVES ABOUT TO SNAP, MY DAUGHTER AND I SAT
in the hallway on the eleventh floor of the great New York
Hospital–Cornell Medical Center and waited for word
from the operating room below, where my wife was
undergoing open-heart surgery. It was the day—June 28,
1974—when we were to find out at last whether modern
surgery could save a life very dear to us, or lose it.

Like most Americans, we had been conditioned to
put our faith in the surgical miracle, to put our trust in
the deft hands of preeminent surgeons now able to go
into the chest cavity and operate upon the heart itself—
now able, God willing, to excise my wife's failing mitral
valve and replace it with a plastic one that would give her
long years of health. This operation, to us, was the only
crisis. Like most Americans, we had no conception of the
further reality, no appreciation of a fundamental fact:
that the surgery itself is often only the first in a long
chain of crises; that, before we were done, we would be
given a full postgraduate course in the strange and terrifying labyrinth that is the medical system.

As we would learn much too late, it is a system so
overburdened, so chaotic, so fragmented—especially so
fragmented—that life-and-death details become lost in

the maze. It is a system in which each expert is a law unto himself in his own special field; a system in which, all too frequently, one expert fails to hold any rational communication with another—and the patient is left in fatal limbo between the two. It is a system that makes little attempt to join sophisticated surgery with postoperative care. It is a system that places undue emphasis on the correctional procedure and pays scant attention to the new and potentially lethal problems that procedure may create. In a medical world so splintered and so insensitive to the whole patient, tragedies occur much too frequently, and the legion of unnumbered, needless dead mock the surgical skills designed to save them.

All this we would learn in time, but that long afternoon while we waited for the surgical verdict, while minutes dragged endlessly into hours, we were taut with the anxiety of ultimate confrontation. Seventeen years of worry lay behind that moment; seventeen years of treating my wife's damaged heart valve with medication, of periodic crises with threatening bronchial illnesses, of repeated hospitalizations, of catheterization tests to see how the damaged valve was functioning; seventeen years of mounting physical and psychological pressures as the heart gradually weakened and life became more of a daily ordeal. It had all come down to this—this moment of time in the operating room with the dread of death and the hope of recovery.

Julia and I had celebrated our thirty-eighth wedding anniversary on June 5. It had not been much of a celebration this time, for over the day had hung the dark cloud of the decision she had made. Dr. Paul A. Ebert, chief of the Department of Surgery at New York–Cornell, had advised my wife that she could wait no longer, that the delay of a year would drastically reduce her chances. A tall, rail-thin man with a kindly face and soft-spoken manner, Dr. Ebert had instilled in Julia a kind of instant trust; and she, impressed, cheered by all she had heard of New York–Cornell as one of the nation's greatest hospitals, had made the almost instantaneous decision to put her life in his hands—to take the gamble that we had dreaded for so long and had known for so long would someday become inevitable.

Now my daughter, Barbara, and I sat at the end of a long hallway leading to the elevator bank and, past that, to the nurses' station. A gray-haired man in bathrobe and slippers came out of one of the semiprivate rooms opening to the hall. A long surgical scar showed above the open neck of his pajama top and ran, as we knew it must, down the center of his chest to the base of the rib cage. A heart-operation patient who had survived, one who had made it.

We knew that Julia's operation would probably take some five hours; we knew there could hardly be any word this soon—and yet we could not sit still in our anxiety to know what was happening in the operating room below us. We had each brought a book to read, but a book was no help. Read a few lines. Look up. Watch a busy nurse bustling down the hall, popping into first one room, then another. Read another few lines. Look up. The words made no sense; the mind wouldn't focus.

Unable to sit still any longer, we would get up, pace down the hall, look inquiringly at the young black woman on duty at the nurses' station. Any word yet? She shakes her head.

Back down the hall. Sit again. Hours of this. And then at 2:45 P.M. the nurse from the desk comes down the hall to go into an adjacent room. She sees us, pauses, and says, "It's all over."

"Is she all right?"

She nods. "They're just cleaning up. They'll be bringing her up in a few minutes."

Relief. God, what relief! Julia had made it. The air whooshed out of our lungs in huge, simultaneous sighs, the first reaction. Then came the second: the wondering, the doubt. How well had she come through that brutal operation? Had she just barely made it? Or had she *really* made it? When could we see Dr. Ebert? When could we know?

Go back down the hall again and talk to the young coordinator at the junction with a crossing hall that leads, on the right, to the women's section, and on the left, to the intensive care unit. "Dr. Ebert is terribly busy," he says, "but I'll try to get someone from the cardiology team to talk to you."

I pace back and rejoin my daughter. More minutes pass; then the elevator down the hall opens. My wife is wheeled out; her attendants swing her quickly to the left, and she vanishes down the other hall into intensive care. We wait again.

Another half, three-quarters of an hour go by, and I go back to talk to the coordinator. He's trying to get someone to tell us how everything went. In the meantime, the X-ray technician hurries down the hall and goes into intensive care to take pictures of my wife's new heart valve, to double-check on how it is functioning.

My daughter and I wait some more. Relatives of other patients come and go. The hall begins to look deserted. And still we sit. Some two hours have passed since the surgery ended, and no one has found the time to talk to us. It was the first indication, we would conclude later, of one of the insidious dangers inherent in modern medical specialization—the fragmentation of care.

4

"That has always struck me," my daughter says now, "as the first illustration we had of this modern, cold, conveyor-belt attitude. The technicians in the operating room had done their job; she was off their assembly line, out of their hands, and it was now up to somebody else. And they obviously couldn't have cared less. All right, Dr. Ebert as chief of the department was understandably too busy to see us. But do you mean to tell me that *nobody* on that cardiology team could have taken five minutes—that was all it would have taken—to tell us how it had gone? What struck me at the time was that feeling I got of lack of concern for the patient, lack of compassion. She wasn't their problem anymore; let somebody else handle it."

The short, stocky X–ray technician, having developed his plates, went hurrying back into intensive care. Some minutes later, the young coordinator, returning from the intensive care unit, saw us still sitting there, realized evidently that no one had yet told us anything, and gestured to us.

"Come on," he said. "I'll take you into intensive care. You can see her now."

My wife lay there, slightly elevated in the bed, sprouting tubes. A tracheal tube was taped to her mouth, and a large plastic tube, running up under the covers into her incision, bubbled away with traces of blood draining from her surgical wound.

Barbara stood close to her mother, touched her arm, and spoke to her.

"Mom," she said, "everything is all right. Dad and I are here."

We did not know if the message would penetrate the fog of anesthesia. Barbara repeated it, and as she did Julia began to shake her head back and forth vigorously, her brows knitting in a frown that deepened rapidly into a dark scowl as if she were saying to herself: "What the hell have they done to me?" As her head-shaking continued, I became alarmed that she might dislodge some of the life-supporting tubes attached to her; but Barbara, who had worked for a time in an operating room in one of our local New Jersey hospitals, knew better than I the significance of what we were seeing and was highly encouraged by it.

"Don't worry, Dad," she said. "That's good. She's coming out of it quickly. She's fighting it. She has a lot of strength."

We turned away from the bed, and the coordinator introduced us to the tall, red-haired resident in charge of the intensive care unit. I told him we hadn't been able to learn any details about the operation. What could he tell us?

"Oh, she's fine," he said. "I know you're probably shocked to see the way she looks right now, but we get many in here who are much worse than she is."

"Just how well has she come through it?" I wanted to know.

"Well, the X rays show the new valve is working perfectly. She had much less bleeding than is customary; they had to use only four units of blood." He smiled at us, kindly, reassuringly.

"The surgeons are very pleased," he said softly. "And so I guess we should be, too, shouldn't we?"

Comforted, relieved, Barbara and I left the great hospital where everything had gone so miraculously well. We boarded our train for the Jersey shore and collapsed in our seats, completely bushed by the strain of the day. We felt as if some unseen hand had unraveled the nervous strands of our beings; but at the time, sweeping through us despite our exhaustion, was a tide of sheer euphoria.

Julia had made it. She had been given a new life. The future would be wonderful, for the great crisis had passed; she had survived the surgical ordeal in marvelous physical shape. And nothing could go wrong now.

2

MY WIFE IS NOW DEAD. SHE SHOULD NOT BE, BUT SHE IS.

She has joined the legion of people who die needlessly, because the surgery that should have given her long years of good health was wasted through failures on virtually every level of the medical system. Her experience was by no means unique; it was not even especially unusual, as the many infinitely sad stories that now clog my files attest. To publicize a tragedy such as hers is to lance a public boil. You are inundated with letters and phone calls, an overwhelming gush of anguish that tells you: "It happened to us, too."

Husbands and wives, sons and daughters are left most miserably bereft, deprived even of the comfort of knowing it was inevitable, haunted by the knowledge that it need not have happened. To come to terms with inevitable death is not easy, but it can be done; to come to terms with the horror of what need never have happened is all but impossible. The survivors are hounded by a hundred "ifs": "if" we had only known, "if" the hospital employees and the doctor had only done their jobs, "if" we, the survivors, had only done something more. "If" we had not put such complete trust in the experts and the system, "if" we had questioned, argued, protested, insisted, screamed for help and attention—done any of these things—he or she would still be alive.

No one knows how many Julia Cooks die unnecessarily each year, for no statistics are kept on the toll taken by sheer neglect. As Dr. George A. Silver, professor of public health at Yale University Medical School, wrote in reply to a letter of mine after Julia's death:

> The points you make in your sad letter, derived from your experience during your wife's illness, are probably not uncommon. Since the kind of record-keeping that would enable the patient to develop valid statistical bases for any conclusion is lacking, I can't say how common these events are. However, it is perfectly plain that in a disorganized medical care system the inadequacy of communications would account for just the kind of results that you report. . . . All I can offer you is the apology of a physician whose colleagues have failed over the years to provide an organized, painstakingly oriented system of medical practice. I've spoken out but obviously that's not enough.

What follows is, of necessity, largely a personal story, though the experiences of many others will enter into it before I am done. It is written not to mourn my wife, but in the hope that the detailing of her experience may stir the conscience of the medical profession on the one hand, and, on the other, alert potential patients to pitfalls in the system and prevent what happened to her from happening to them. To accomplish these ends, even in part, it is necessary to tell Julia's story in step-by-step fashion, using hers as the individual case that illustrates innumerable others. Only by looking at it in detail can one see what happened, how it happened, why it happened—and how, hopefully, such tragedies may be avoided.

I like to remember Julia as she was when I met her in late December, 1933—a tall, lissome girl, graceful of figure, with the sunniest of dispositions. One of life's eternal optimists, she seemed to embody Robert Browning's favorite dictum: "God's in his heaven—All's right with the world." She had a whacky, delightful sense of humor, and I called her my "monkey" and my "minx." And, of course, we went on from there, as lovers have since the beginning of time, to fashion other terms of endearment precious only to ourselves.

Chronic illness over the years dimmed the sunniness of her personality, but many of the basic traits that so endeared her to me never changed. She was the kind of person of whom my mother could say, after knowing her for forty years, "I never heard her say an unkind word about anyone." She was the most unselfish person I have ever known. As her niece told me after her death, "I think Aunt Julie had the biggest heart of anyone I've ever met." When we had an anniversary or she had a birthday and I was at a loss as to what to get her, I would sometimes give her a check and say: "Now I want you to spend this on yourself. Get something you *really* want with it." She never would; the money always went to buy something she thought her children or grandchildren needed.

She was not the kind of woman who wanted expensive jewelry or a mink coat or a $300 dress. She was the kind who enjoyed the beauty of a glorious sunset, who liked to rise early and marvel at the golden glow of the sun rising out of the sea, who delighted to eat breakfast with me in the stern of our outboard boat as it rocked gently at its dock in the marina while ducks quacked and foraged for food in the shallows by the marshes.

With it all, she had a lot of courage. I will never forget the time in 1950 when she made the same kind of discovery that so many women have made. She discovered a lump in her left breast, and it was quite large by the time she became aware of it. Our family doctor and the surgeon to whom he sent her were both alarmed; from the size and feel of it, they were fearful it was cancer.

But Julia appeared unconcerned; at least, if she worried, she took great care that neither I nor the children should get the faintest hint of it. Fred and Barbara were small then, and Julia, careful to reassure them, marched off to the hospital as if she faced nothing more serious than a tonsillectomy.

"Don't worry," I remember her telling the children. "Everything is going to be all right. Mother's just going to the hospital for a couple of days, and then I'll be back and we'll all be together again. There's nothing to worry about."

I never admired her more. And the result vindicated her courage and her optimism; the large lump turned out to be a cyst, not the thing we had dreaded.

Marked and sad was the contrast between that woman and the one who entered New York–Cornell for open-heart surgery in 1974. Chronic illness had taken its emotional and psychological toll. Her heart problem at the time it developed was not something to be cured by a quick remedy, but a burden that she would have to carry every day, every month, every year, knowing that, in all probability, death lay at the end of the ordeal. I suppose that for a supreme optimist like her the burden had to be especially heavy. Suddenly the "all's right with the world" faith that had sustained her ceased to have any validity, and she became with the passing years terribly depressed and in the end almost neurotic about her condition.

Hers was a common enough ailment and a common enough reaction. Seventeen years is a long time to live with such a burden, and heart patients who have to carry their load for so long frequently develop psychological problems.

Apparently Julia's heart trouble, as is true in many cases, stemmed from a bout with rheumatic fever when she was a child. She had no recollection of the illness, but it had left her with what was called at the time a "heart murmur." She was not allowed to take physical training in her latter years in high school; but her physician apparently felt that youth would cure all, and no one explained to her how serious that "murmur" might become in the years ahead.

In the optimism of our youth, the existence of this vague potential problem had not disturbed us. Julia was a strong person physically; she had a lot of stamina. I might drag along with a cold for a couple of weeks; she would throw off the same bug in a few days. She could swim tirelessly and play Ping-Pong until she literally wore me out. How were we to suspect that her "heart murmur" would develop into a life-threatening weakness?

But age, increasing weight, and the strains of childbirth all took their toll; and when Julia was forty-six, her mitral valve (the large valve on the left side of the heart that controls the flow of blood to the lungs) began to give her trouble. In the chill weather of that long-ago fall of 1957, she developed a hard, hacking cough; and it was in the treatment of this that we encountered the first of the series of medical blunders that were to pursue us relentlessly through the years until the last of them finally took her life.

Much has been written about the inadequacies of American medical care in the ghettos and in deprived rural areas where there are not enough doctors and the few hospitals are substandard and poorly staffed. Our experience took place in a different kind of area, one with supposedly good medical care available. The Asbury Park region where we lived, on the Jersey coast, had at the onset of Julia's illness two large, fully accredited hospitals; it was a prosperous suburban area, its economy nourished by large nearby military bases, and it had more supposedly well-trained, board-accredited physicians in various specialties than many sections of the nation.

Our family doctor had been recommended to me by one of the executives of the newspaper for which I worked; he was a general practitioner with a flourishing practice and a good reputation. He had delivered our daughter and treated our family for a variety of ailments over the years, and he knew all about Julia's "heart murmur." Yet when she went to him with her troublesome cough, he ignored the possibility of a heart problem and decided that she must have a cold and that she simply needed an injection.

The shots that he gave her had no effect. The cough persisted; indeed, it became more wracking. Yet the doctor continued to believe that Julia had a cold; the true nature of her problem never occurred to him.

A medical expert to whom, after her death, I described this early sequence, shook his head in impatient disgust. "With a cough like that," he said, "one of the first things you should think of is a possible heart involvement. All right, granting that at first he thought it was a cold, still when she kept returning to him over a six-week period as you say she did, he should not have kept right on pounding down the same trail. He should have considered other possibilities."

Our doctor, however, did not. We would wonder afterward whether the damage to her heart would have been so severe without the initial mistake. If her condition had been diagnosed accurately and treated promptly, could she have had a longer and better life? That is just one of the imponderables. We will never know.

Dissatisfied with her treatment and increasingly worried, I wanted her to change doctors, but she would not. This was characteristic of Julia. She was an intensely loyal person, loyal to her family, her friends, and unfortunately to her doctor. She seemed to feel that it would be almost an act of betrayal to seek another opinion.

And so there came a night later that year, somewhere around Thanksgiving time, when she staggered into the house from choir practice at the First Presbyterian Church. She just made it through the front door into our vestibule and collapsed there, leaning against the wall.

"I can't breathe," she gasped.

That was the first of many panics.

3

JULIA WAS LYING COLLAPSED IN BED WHEN THE NEW doctor called. He was a younger physician and bore a family name long respected in medical circles in our area. Though a general practitioner, he had devoted special attention to the study and treatment of heart cases. Through his stethoscope, he listened to the sounds of Julia's laboring heart and at once recognized her problem.

"Did you have rheumatic fever when you were young?" he asked her. She told him she had no recollection of it.

"Well, you did," he told her. "There isn't any doubt about it; it was fairly common in this area."

He explained to Julia that what she had always regarded as an unimportant "heart murmur" had now become a damaged mitral valve that was restricting the flow of blood from the left side of her heart. Hers was a problem, as we later learned, that often overtakes "heart murmur" victims when they get into their forties and the physical system begins to feel the wear of years. Digitalis, a drug that stimulates and improves the action of the heart, is the recognized medication for the problem, and our new doctor put Julia on a digitalis compound immediately.

"When you are better," he said, "I want you to come into my office and have a cardiogram. The digitalis will help you, but there is always more that can be done. They are now doing heart operations for problems like yours with great success, you know."

That was the first mention of the ultimate prospect that was to haunt our remaining years together.

Julia responded well to digitalis medication. She seemed to have almost as much energy as usual in the mornings; and when she began to tire after lunch, she followed her new doctor's advice and took a nap for an hour or two. The rest seemed to revive her, and she would cook dinner and finish her household chores as usual.

New problems kept developing, however. My wife's heart was now fibrillating; in other words, its muscle fibers were contracting irregularly. In an effort to restore it to a regular beat, our new doctor prescribed quinidine. Unfortunately, Julia was allergic to this old drug, for which no effective substitute had yet been found, and she had to be taken off the medication. She had to resign herself to living the rest of her life with an uneven, uncertain heartbeat.

More scary were the intermittent mysterious attacks that she now suffered. When these came on, Julia's face would pale, her forehead would break out in a clammy sweat, and her erratic pulse would fade to almost nothing. These spells were never of long duration; they passed over before we could get in touch with our busy doctor or before he could get to our house. He never did manage to arrive in time to catch Julia in the midst of such an alarming performance, and so he had no opportunity to make an accurate diagnosis. (Later doctors would theorize that Julia had probably had a blood clot somewhere in her system and that these strange attacks were precipitated by small bits of it flaking off. If one had hit a vital organ, it could have killed her.)

After our new physician had examined Julia thoroughly, no further mention was made of the possibility of open-heart surgery. A major deterrent was her weight. She had been a slim 132 pounds when we were married in 1936, but with the years her weight had soared; it was around 180 when her heart trouble developed. Tall, at five feet eight, she carried the weight well, and she was still graceful and attractive; but that excess poundage represented a deadly hazard if open-heart surgery became necessary.

Our doctor told Julia frankly that she probably could not live more than five to eight years unless she got rid of those excess pounds; and I, horrified at the imminence of death he suggested, kept arguing with my wife about her weight problem, emphasizing that she *had* to stay on a diet.

It was a losing battle. To do Julia justice, shedding weight was abnormally difficult for her. She had a slight thyroid problem that had developed after her first pregnancy, and this could not be treated medically because medication to help the thyroid would have adversely affected the heart. And so the combination of her thyroid imbalance and her gradually lessening physical activity handicapped her in the attempt to slough off the necessary number of pounds. She could eat an amazingly small amount of food and still not lose; then, becoming discouraged, she would act like a drunkard falling off the wagon and go on a brief eating binge. Remorseful, she would try to get back on her diet, a regimen not easily reestablished once the chain of habit was broken. Thus it went for years; Julia would lose three pounds, gain back two, then struggle to lose those two all over again.

Despite all this—despite those alarming and mysterious attacks, despite the battle of the diet and the apprehension about her condition—those first years were not too difficult. Julia was still active in the home, and she retained much of her natural cheeriness and optimism. She was always at her best when some crisis arose in the family, or when one or another of us needed her support.

I will never forget the night in late November, 1959, when I came home from New York, fired from my newspaper job after a tangle with management over charges of municipal corruption I had made on a television program. I was hurt, bitterly angry about what I felt had been a callous and unjustified stand by the paper; but the first thing I saw when I got off the train was Julia driving up in our car and greeting me with her usual warm, welcoming smile. Her first words to me were: "Don't worry. Everything is going to be all right."

I asked her if she knew all that had happened.

"I know," she said. "The phone has been ringing all afternoon; people are on your side. You're going to be better off than you've ever been before. Now you can do what you've always wanted to do; you can stay home and do your writing."

As it turned out, she was right, but I could not know that then. All I knew was that I was thankful to have such a wife, one who offered not a word of criticism or reproach, but faced the uncertain future with such confidence in me and such morale-boosting optimism.

The relatively good time continued for five more years. Shadowing our lives was the worry about Julia's condition, a chronic ailment that would never get better; but we lived in reasonable thankfulness that, for the time being, it seemed no worse. My wife was well enough to travel with me when I left home to research magazine articles and books. Though as a free lance I often found myself working seven days a week, we managed on a cou-

ple of rare occasions to wedge in brief vacations in Little-
ton, New Hampshire, in the heart of the White Moun-
tains that we loved. I no longer had to work and commute
twelve to fourteen hours a day; we had the time to be
together, and this to us, still in love after all the years, was
a boon indeed.

Julia had defied and defeated that five-year predic-
tion of doom and seemed well on her way to outliving the
eight-year forecast, though she had not been able to lose
the amount of weight her doctor thought she should.
Then, abruptly, in the summer of 1964, we reached a
turning point in her struggle for life. Our experience
with hospitals began, and the slow disintegration of a
personality began with it.

4

It was a Saturday afternoon in late June, hot
and humid in Washington, D.C. Julia and I had spent
nearly three weeks in the capital and were winding up
research for a short book that I would have less than two
months to write. We had enjoyed the break in the normal
routine of our days; our hotel room was air-conditioned
and comfortable, and Julia was in good spirits.

Early in my writing career, she had typed all my
manuscripts, for she was a fast and accurate typist. After
the onset of her heart trouble, she had given this up because the constant movement of her hands upon the keys
exhausted her. This time, however, she had been feeling
so well that she insisted on typing some notes for me
while I waded through the texts of speeches, a variety of
transcripts, and mounds of clippings. The work did not
seem to tire her.

We went out to lunch and returned to our hotel to
spend a leisurely afternoon, napping, reading a little,
enjoying the opportunity to loaf now that our work was
almost finished. We would be driving back to New Jersey
Monday morning.

This pleasant prospect was suddenly shattered when,
in mid-afternoon, Julia suffered the most violent of those
mysterious attacks that had so alarmed us in recent years.

This time, however, in addition to the usual symptoms—the cold, clammy sweat and the fading pulse—she was sick to her stomach, retching in great, wracking heaves in our bathroom. I thought that she must be having a major heart attack and phoned a panicked SOS to the hotel desk clerk. He summoned help, and soon Dr. George T. Economos, a heart specialist on the staff of George Washington University Hospital, came to our room.

He examined Julia carefully and allayed my major worry. "I don't know just what it is," I remember him telling me, "but I'm certain of one thing: it's not a heart attack, and she's in no immediate danger. But she is very ill, and we'll have to get her into the hospital to make some tests. Do you want me to call an ambulance or will you take her?"

He assured me it would be safe for me to drive her to the hospital in our car; and Julia, shying from creating a sensation by summoning an ambulance, wanted me to take her. The hospital was only a few blocks away, and I drove up to the emergency entrance, where attendants, already alerted by Dr. Economos, met us with a wheelchair and whisked my wife away for a cardiogram and heart X ray.

I made arrangements for her admittance and waited until she was brought to her semiprivate room. Afterward —something that greatly disturbed her—she had no recollection of what had happened until she found herself in bed with me standing beside her. She must have been practically out on her feet when I took her to the hospital, for her mind was a blank about everything that had happened just after she arrived.

When I saw her the next morning, the change was remarkable. She appeared fully recovered and in the best of spirits, sitting up in bed bright-eyed, smiling, buoyant. It was wonderful to see her so miraculously restored, and

I had no doubt that she could go home with me on Monday.

By late afternoon, when I saw her again, the picture had changed radically. She lay back in bed, collapsed and weak. Alarmed, I tried to find out what had happened, and Dr. Economos told me that, as part of the effort to track down the cause of her mysterious seizure, they had taken her off all medications to see how she would react. The result, it would seem, should have been entirely predictable. To take a patient whose heart had been sustained by digitalis for seven years off the medication would seem guaranteed to produce just this kind of collapse.

Afterward, with the benefit of hindsight, I would plague myself with the first of those many "ifs" that still harrow me. What would have happened if I had rebelled, if I had not gone along with the "experts" but had insisted on immediate resumption of digitalis? What if I had taken my wife home with me the next day even though I had to sign her out myself? One can never know the answers to such questions, but of one thing I am certain: what followed in the next long weeks had a destructive psychological effect on her.

At the time, the experts at the hospital were absorbed only by the physical mystery. What had caused that violent Saturday afternoon attack? They would need time and would have to run a series of tests to find out. This seemed logical; and so it became obvious that I would have to leave Julia behind when I left on Monday.

This meant that I would be abandoning her away from home, in a strange city, but it could not be helped. Our livelihood depended upon my writing, and I had a deadline that it was imperative to meet. Some deadlines are not so rigid that they cannot be bent a bit in an emergency; but this, unfortunately, was not one of those. I was caught in a time bind, and I had to get back to my desk. Anyway, I reasoned, Julia would not have to stay long, just long enough for some tests; surely I could bring her back home in a week.

I talked to her daily by telephone, and she was quite impressed by the thoroughness of the tests she was given, by the way the hospital cardiology team thronged around her bed. But as the days crept into weeks, it seemed to me that little progress was being made.

We in the family did our best to keep in touch. Barbara drove down to Washington to spend a day with her mother. Another time our son, Fred, went down to see her and came back alarmed, having found his mother in a state of collapse. It developed that the hospital, unwilling to take anyone's word that Julia was allergic to quinidine, had tested her reaction to the drug, producing the frightening result my son had witnessed. Worried by all this, I abandoned my work and went to Washington to see my wife and find out what the devil was going on.

A major effort, I learned, was being aimed at Julia's weight problem. She had been placed first on a 1,000-calorie-a-day diet—and hadn't lost an ounce. Not until her intake was reduced to a miniscule 800 calories a day did she begin to lose. This was fine as far as it went, but what about the major issue—the heart problem? Dr. Economos said that there was one procedure the hospital staff thought might help: an electric-shock treatment that might convert my wife's heart to a normal, regular rhythm. When our doctor in Asbury Park learned of this, he snorted in disgust.

"The trouble with some of these Goddamned university hospitals," he said, "is that they like guinea pigs for their students to practice on. What's the point of doing this? Even if they succeed in restoring Julia's heart to a normal rhythm, they can't keep it that way without quinidine—and she's allergic to quinidine."

That, I have to believe, was simple common sense. And so again, looking back, I am harried by one of those "ifs." I was impressed by our doctor's logic at the time. Why, then, did I let my wife go ahead with the experiment? Largely, I suppose, because she wanted to try it. She had been so impressed by the staff at George Washington that she believed they must know best. Perhaps I should have argued the issue with her; perhaps I didn't because I, too, was inclined to put more trust in the cardiology team of a great hospital than in the opinion of a local doctor who was not even a board-certified cardiologist.

Years later and much too late, I would conclude that the patient and the patient's family have to double-check the experts, have to use their own common sense and good judgment in such situations instead of putting blind faith in the professionals. But at the time none of us had learned this hard lesson, and we decided to let the hospital go ahead. Julia came home for nearly three weeks, from the last part of July to the beginning of August. She had to take Coumadin, a blood-thinning drug, before the great attempt could be made to regulate her heartbeat, and this medication could be taken just as effectively at home as in the hospital.

In early August, her blood appropriately thinned out, she returned to George Washington for the electric-shock treatment. It didn't work. Her heart continued to fibrillate, and the outcome dealt her the first of those psychic shocks that were to be so destructive.

She had built her hopes high. She had been so impressed by the innumerable tests she had been given, the meticulous care, the sophisticated daily examinations, that she had come to place an almost mystic faith in the great hospital and its staff. Surely they were going to help her. Even though the electric-shock treatment could not correct her mitral-valve impairment, the restoration of her heart to a normal rhythm would make her feel miraculously better. So she reasoned. And then she woke to the knowledge of complete failure.

She cried brokenly, in despair, and was comforted by a Chinese woman physician on the cardiology team. The doctor tried to assure her that all was not hopeless, that she was no worse off than before, that she could still live a good and useful life. It was a sympathetic and compassionate effort for which Julia was always grateful, but in the light of subsequent events I have to think its impact was slight. The psychological damage had been done.

In this state, my wife left George Washington University Hospital. The results of her six-week hospital confinement seemed to me minimal. The 800-calorie regimen had brought her weight down to 159 pounds. Digoxin, a more effective form of digitalis, had been substituted for the compound she had been taking, and one new medication had been added—Bicillin, a long-lasting form of penicillin, administered as a protection for her heart and lungs against infection. And that was it.

What caused that violent Saturday afternoon attack in our hotel room? Despite all their tests, the hospital experts never could pinpoint the cause. As time went on, however, it became clear to us that, in this respect at least, there had been a decided change for the better in my wife's condition. She never had another of those alarming attacks, and this fact subsequently led our cardiologist to theorize that the Washington episode had been triggered by the last of a blood clot breaking loose. Luckily, if that was the case, the clot had passed through her stomach without touching any vital organ.

Before my wife returned home, I discussed her condition at length with Dr. Economos. She had been examined from the hair of her head to the tip of her toes, and she was in excellent physical shape except for the one thing that mattered most, her heart. The outlook there was pretty bleak, wasn't it? I asked him.

"Well, not necessarily," he told me. "Look at it this way: considering the condition of her valve, her age, her weight, she should not be as well as she is. All I can say is that her heart must be compensating in some way that we have not been able to determine; and so, if she is careful and keeps her weight down, who knows? She could go on for a long while."

I wondered whether the fact that I had started giving my wife vitamin E about a year after her heart trouble developed had something to do with her inexplicably better condition. Canadian doctors had issued enthusiastic reports about the efficacy of vitamin E in treating heart problems, but the American medical profession took the stand that the vitamin was virtually worthless. Dr. Economos doubted it had helped my wife, but had no objection to her continuing to take it; at least, he said, it could do no harm. He also warned me that the time would eventually come when Julia would have to risk open-heart surgery, but for the present that certainly wasn't advisable.

In a final conversation with both my wife and myself, he tried to impress upon Julia the importance of her weight. If she could continue to lose, if she really got her weight down, she would feel much better and her chances of living longer would be greatly improved. Then he delivered a warning, necessary in the circumstances, but one that, added to the failed electric-shock experiment, increased Julia's apprehensions. He explained that the impaired mitral valve decreased the flow of blood through the lungs and that, if Julia caught a cold, there was always danger that pneumonia might develop.

"Get in touch with your doctor as soon as a cold starts," I recall him saying, "and try to treat it quickly with antibiotics to prevent more serious complications."

It was, I am sure, sound medical advice, but to my wife it was scary. She came out of the long summer in the hospital, where she had received care and attention such as she had never had before, not only with high hopes unfulfilled but with new burdens. She became a much-changed person. The optimism with which she had sailed through life, with which until now she had coped even with her heart problem, was virtually destroyed.

About a month after her return home, in September of 1964, she contracted a cold and at once collapsed into bed, moaning and crying, "I feel as if I'm going to die." She had never acted this way in all our previous years together; but now each time she got a cold, she went into an emotional tailspin, and the despairing cry, "I feel awful, I think I'm going to die," became a constant refrain during the next ten years.

5

In the summer of 1965, we came to another critical turning point. Julia began to wheeze with almost every breath she took. She went to her doctor, the one who, in my judgment at least, had been so correct in frowning on the electric-shock experiment; and he dismissed her new symptoms almost casually.

"You've got cardiac asthma," he told her. "Get yourself an asthmatic inhaler."

Julia got the inhaler, but continued to wheeze. It seemed to me that the inhaler, while it might ease the symptoms and help her to breathe, wasn't getting at the root of her new and disturbing trouble. "Why not see another doctor?" I suggested. Julia, with her stubborn sense of loyalty, balked at the idea. Even though she realized that the inhaler wasn't doing her much good, she wouldn't consider a change of physicians.

Fortunately, in midsummer, her doctor took the first real vacation he had had in years, going to Europe with his wife. In his absence, Julia's wheezing seemed to become worse. It became obvious even to her that something more had to be done.

We had been close friends with another couple ever since the early days of our marriage. The other wife had worked for years as a receptionist and medical secretary in doctors' offices and knew the reputations of all the cardiologists in our area. We consulted her, and she gave me a list of three prominent specialists. Though she avoided making any specific recommendation, it was obvious to me from what she said that there was one she regarded most highly—a man whom I shall refer to here only as The Great Doctor.

He certainly lived the role. If a casting director had sought a prototype for the supreme egos of the profession, he could have made no better selection. Tall, handsome, a distinguished bit of gray beginning to streak his hair, he would come swinging into his office, whistling a popular show tune and making some jocular comment about the number of patients waiting to present him with their problems.

During the years we knew him, he rose steadily in professional esteem until he became chief of the Department of Medicine, virtually chief of staff, of the largest regional hospital in our Monmouth County area. He relished every bit of his authority and lived his role to the hilt. He strode the halls of his hospital like a demigod. When he ordered something, nurses flew; when he walked into a staff conference, an awed hush fell over the room as lesser mortals waited for his words.

He was a board-certified internist and cardiologist; he was a specially qualified expert who spent hours double-checking cardiograms taken in the hospital to make certain that subtle warning signs were not missed. From every standpoint, his professional qualifications seemed to guarantee my wife the best of care; and when we first met him in 1965, he impressed both of us with his knowledge and competence. He gave Julia a fluoroscopic examination, then revealed what he'd found.

"You have congestive heart failure," he told my wife. "There is fluid building up around the heart, and this is what is causing your wheezing. I'll have to put you in the hospital for a few days to get rid of it."

We were both startled by this, not having anticipated the necessity of hospitalization. And both of us were haunted, I think, by the memory of the previous summer's long stay in George Washington. He evidently saw this and tried to reassure us.

"It won't be long, probably just a couple of days," he said, "But we've got to get rid of that fluid and see what we can do about keeping your chest and lungs clear."

Jocularly, he told my wife, who always had such a blooming complexion that few, meeting her, ever suspected she had a health problem: "You certainly don't look like somebody needing hospitalization, but I'm afraid you do. I'd like to put you in the hospital this afternoon and get going on this right away"

Our heads reeling from the suddenness, we returned home, packed the nightgowns and accessories my wife would need, and went back to have her admitted to the hospital. The Great Doctor proved as good as his word. This time, her stay was short, only three days as I recall, and much was accomplished in that brief time.

A diuretic administered the day she was admitted got rid of the threatening fluid, and The Great Doctor increased her medication in the hope of preventing a new buildup. He explained to me: "I've increased her digoxin from twenty-five milligrams to fifty a day, and I think we can keep her clear on that. But I want you to understand that this is just about the maximum dosage we can give. There isn't any leeway. If we can stabilize her with this— and I think we can—she should be all right. But she'll be very finely poised; if anything else develops, we'll be in trouble."

I told him I understood.

"Good," he said. "Let's not worry about that now.

Her chest is clear, and you can take her home tomorrow. Let's just hope for the best and see how it goes."

The Great Doctor's program of increased medication worked. Julia's wheezing stopped; fluoroscopic examination, once a month at first, then once every two months as her condition remained stable, showed that her chest was beautifully clear. The Great Doctor, it seemed, had done more for my wife than had any of her earlier physicians or the experts with whom she had spent the previous summer. She often said, "I might have died if I had kept on using that inhaler and hadn't gone to him." It was the beginning of her unalterable faith in The Great Doctor; she felt that he had pulled her back from the brink.

She was also reassured by the care he took in explaining her condition to her; she got, I think, a clearer picture than she had ever had of the nature and complications of her problem. In her first long consultation with the doctor after she left the hospital, he described for her the considerable enlargement of the right side of her heart.

What had happened was roughly this: Though the mitral valve is located on the left side of the heart, it handles the return flow of blood from the right side. The heart has two ventricles or pumps. The left has the toughest job, thrusting blood at high pressure through the large aortic valve, the main trunkline for the entire body. The right ventricle has the easier task of sending blood on a much shorter journey through the lungs. This blood then returns through the pulmonary veins to the mitral valve where it is received and passes on into the left ventricle to be pumped out again through the aorta. When the mitral valve is impaired, this smooth flow of blood is impeded, and a kind of backwash is created. Since the left ventricle has the hardest pumping job, nature has made its muscular walls much thicker and tougher than those of its companion right-hand pump. However, a mitral-valve malfunction puts an increased pressure into the pulmonary tree, and this in turn puts a disproportionate strain on the thinner-walled right ventricle which, in struggling to perform its task, bulges and becomes enlarged.

Julia's heart enlargement was, therefore, not unnatural. In describing this to her, the doctor told her not to worry; such enlargements were the inevitable by-product of mitral-valve malfunction, and hers was not as bad as it might have been, not as bad as many.

Julia left his office in a much more cheerful frame of mind, convinced that she had really found a doctor who knew what he was doing and was capable of helping her. Her more optimistic attitude was reflected that night when our son's mother-in-law telephoned to find out what she had learned from this first long talk with her new heart expert. Julia replied with one of those fey flashes of humor so characteristic of her.

"Well," she quipped, "he found out that I am all heart."

6

Julia's weight remained a serious problem. Despite Dr. Economos's frank counsel, despite the hope he held out to her for a longer life if she continued to reduce, she just couldn't do it. It would have taken grim determination, given Julia's handicaps, for her to have kept on a rigid diet that would have removed the necessary pounds; and my wife, lovable person that she was, unfortunately did not have that kind of exceptional willpower.

She tried various regimens, and sometimes she tried hard. She went to Weight Watchers and lost a few pounds, but quickly became sick of the emphasis on seafood. Even here, she was restricted; there were many things that, on account of her heart condition, she could not eat. Shellfish, which she liked, were forbidden because they contain too much sodium; similarly, she could never eat tuna fish or canned products of any kind because of their salt content. Her stomach rebelled at cottage cheese for lunch or broiled flounder for dinner. And so she abandoned Weight Watchers. "I'm their only failure," she would say in humorous disparagement of herself.

For years she recorded her weight faithfully every week on sheets of paper that became testaments to her discouraging struggle. This record shows how her weight crept up again into the 175- to 180-pound range after the George Washington experience, and how it came back to 159 or 160 at the end. The Great Doctor was understandably worried about this aspect of her case. Like every other physician who examined Julia, he was convinced that the day would come when medication would no longer serve—that eventually she would have to risk open-heart surgery. And when that day came could she possibly survive, given the condition of her heart, her age, and her weight?

Even if the answer could have been "Yes," there were other crucial issues to be decided in a case so complex and so delicately balanced. When would be the best time? Should the gamble be taken soon, before advancing age further complicated the situation? Or would it be more prudent to wait, letting Julia get what good she could out of the years, taking the plunge only when there was no alternative?

The Great Doctor weighed all these considerations carefully; and two years after he began examining my wife and evaluating her multiple problems, he decided on a cautious first step. He told us that he wanted to find out two things: the precise condition of Julia's mitral valve, something that could be determined only by a sophisticated test called a catheterization; and, once this information had been obtained, the considered judgment of a leading open-heart surgeon on the feasibility of an operation. He assured Julia that he was not proposing any drastic immediate action; he was merely trying to learn all the facts, to explore the possibilities.

The specialist to whom he sent us was Dr. Charles Bailey, a pioneer in open-heart surgery, who would both perform the catheterization and provide the opinion. Dr. Bailey headed the cardiology team at small, ancient-looking St. Barnabas Hospital in New York's Bronx, and it was there I took my wife in the summer of 1967.

A heart catheterization is a nerve-wracking, exhausting procedure that takes hours. The patient cannot be tranquilized or anesthetized because heart functions must be tested under normal conditions. My wife was placed flat on her back, and a fine catheter was inserted into the vein of one arm at about elbow level. This catheter was then wriggled slowly up the vein, and my wife could follow its progress on a television monitor. It crawled up at a snail's pace until its tip was inserted into the mitral valve of her heart. It is a frightening procedure for a patient to watch.

My wife's mouth became parched, her back ached, and the strain became almost unbearable. Mrs. Bailey, who was there to assist her husband during the procedure, stood over her and bathed her forehead, moistened her lips, and tried to comfort her; but Julia was so exhausted by the time she was brought back to her hospital room that she could barely flutter her eyelids at me. "I'm too tired to talk," she whispered. "I've got to go to sleep. You had better go back home."

Dr. Bailey's subsequent report to The Great Doctor was optimistic. The condition of Julia's mitral valve was not as bad as had been feared, and Dr. Bailey suggested the possibility of using a technique he had perfected to avoid total valve replacement in such cases. His method consisted of taking a piece of tendon from one leg and reinforcing the lip of the valve with it, a procedure he felt would work in Julia's case. His recommendation: operate.

After studying the report, The Great Doctor discussed it with us. "I found out the principal thing I wanted to know," he said. "Dr. Bailey thinks it's safe to operate. But let's not rush into things. Since the condition of the valve is better than we thought it might be, we have time; we don't have to hurry. And before we do anything, I'll want another opinion."

It was a cautious, careful approach, and we liked it. Another fifteen months passed. The Great Doctor continued to examine my wife regularly; and when he went to cardiologists' conventions, he discussed her case with some of the nation's leading specialists. In November, 1968, he decided that the time had come to act.

Dr. John F. Dammann, Jr., of the University of Virginia Hospital in Charlottesville, had the reputation of being one of the country's foremost heart surgeons. He had been praised publicly for his work by Dr. Christiaan Barnard, the South African pioneer who had startled the world with the first successful heart transplant. The Great Doctor had talked with Dr. Dammann. I never knew the details (I was forced to conclude later that the discussion must have been brief and extremely tentative), but our expert cardiologist appeared convinced that this time Julia would get more than just "another opinion"—she would have her operation.

He was sending all her records to Dr. Dammann, he said, and his office would make arrangements for her to be admitted to the University of Virginia Hospital on December 3, 1968. "They will want to examine you first, naturally," he told Julia, "but go down with the idea that you are going to have surgery, for I feel certain you will."

To encourage Julia, he gave her the name and address of another woman patient of his who had been operated on by Dr. Dammann and was back home, feeling well. He suggested that my wife talk to this survivor (which Julia later did), and he advised us to be prepared for about a three-week stay in Virginia.

Breezily, cheerfully, he then dismissed us. "Go and have your heart operation, and I will see you in three weeks," I recall him saying.

Open-heart surgery represents one of the most terrifying and awesome ordeals in medicine. Julia was not as familiar with the details as I was, and I thought it better for her peace of mind that she not know. But of course, being no fool and sometimes almost psychically perceptive, she sensed enough to realize that she was facing a rugged, life-threatening operation.

The procedure, in brief, involves sawing through the sternum, or breastbone, to which the ribs are attached; spreading the ribs wide to expose the heart; freezing the heart into immobility; and turning all bodily functions over to a heart-lung machine that keeps blood and oxygen pumping through the system while a surgical team works on the organ. The procedure is hours long; in Julia's case the surgeons would excise the damaged valve and insert a plastic one. When the operation is finished, an electric shock jolts the heart back into action, and the patient, sprouting a forest of tubes, is rushed into intensive care where bodily functions are monitored minute by minute.

It is a prospect from which anyone might be justified in recoiling, but Julia did not. It was characteristic of her that she might moan and complain that she was dying with a mere cold; but, faced with a major challenge, she met it gallantly. Calmly, she accepted The Great Doctor's advice, and on December 2, 1968, we drove to Charlottesville.

We reported to the hospital as instructed about one o'clock the following afternoon, Julia's bag packed with everything she might need during her three-week stay. I told the woman at the admissions desk that my wife, a patient of Dr. Dammann's, had come to be admitted for heart surgery. The woman searched her records, a baffled look on her face; she could find nothing to indicate that a patient named Julia B. Cook was expected. A minor oversight, no doubt.

"Oh, well," the admissions clerk said, "leave your bag here. You'll have to go down for a heart X ray anyhow, so why don't you do that now?"

We were directed to the lab, where Julia's heart was X-rayed. Then we were told to go to an examining section, where my wife was placed in one of the curtained individual cubicles. I sat outside in the waiting room and waited. And waited.

Other patients, who had arrived after we had, came, were examined, departed. The afternoon passed, and I began to wonder: What has happened to my wife?

Finally, I was summoned into a small consulting room. Dr. Dammann and his aides were there, and so was Julia. I cannot attempt to quote that conversation; surprise and shock must have wiped out memory of the words. What registered was one simple, incredible fact: Dr. Dammann and his staff had known nothing about Julia. They had not been aware she was coming until they found this woman they could not identify stretched out in one of their cubicles awaiting examination.

What about the records The Great Doctor had dispatched? Dr. Dammann had never seen them; he had no idea what could have happened to them.

Offhand, Dr. Dammann said, he did not think he would operate. His first brief examination of Julia had made him doubt that the operation was advisable, but he would want to look further into her case. He would try to get in touch with The Great Doctor and go over the details with him, and he wanted Julia to come back to the hospital the next morning for a series of tests that would help him make a final decision.

We recaptured my wife's suitcase and headed for our motel across the street. Julia was so upset that her mood can only be adequately described as "spitting mad." "I'm never, *never* going to have that damned operation," she raged as we trudged across the street.

She told me that her first indication that something had gone wrong came as she was waiting to be examined. Residents and interns trooped past, examined other patients, and went away, but no one paid any attention to her. Finally, she heard a couple of members of the cardiology team passing her booth, and one said to the other: "Who is that woman in there? Do you know who she is? What is she here for?"

Back in our motel room, I put in a call to The Great Doctor and explained what had happened. Then Julia got on the phone, raving and swearing she would never have the operation. She was not even going back to the hospital the next day—the hell with it. The Great Doctor tried to calm her down and finally persuaded her at least to return for the tests. Still muttering that she wasn't going to have the operation, no matter what, she gave the phone back to me; and The Great Doctor, seemingly much shaken by the episode, promised to rush off duplicates of Julia's records to Dr. Dammann and to talk to him at length by telephone.

We returned to the hospital the next morning, and Dr. Dammann's cardiology team put Julia through a series of exercise tests. "She did very well," one of them told me.

Among other things, the doctors were impressed by Julia's good facial color. Did she use makeup or rouge? No, she told them, she never had; her color was natural.

Dr. Dammann saw us after the examination was completed. He told us flatly that he wouldn't operate. My wife's weight disturbed him. Except in an emergency, he said, he wouldn't operate on Julia unless she lost some 35 pounds and got down to 140. "We have found that we have much more serious postoperative lung problems when we have to operate on persons who are overweight," Dr. Dammann told us. He indicated plainly that he didn't think Julia's chances of survival would be good if she went into surgery with the weight she was carrying.

There were other reasons, sound and logical, for delay. The hospital tests showed that my wife's mitral valve was not so bad that she needed immediate surgery. So why risk it? In addition, Dr. Dammann pointed out, the plastic valves used in such operations were being constantly improved. "The valves we are using today are one hundred percent more efficient than the ones we were using two or three years ago," he said. "And further improvements are being made all the time. The valves we will have in a couple of years will certainly be far superior to those we are using today. So why operate now?"

In conclusion, he came back to the weight problem and gave Julia a stern lecture. If she got rid of those thirty-five pounds, she might not need the operation at all, or at least not for a very long time. And then, if she did have to have it, she would have a far better chance of survival. Her very life, he emphasized, depended on her losing that weight.

We left, visited one of our favorite historic sites—Thomas Jefferson's home at Monticello—and drove home the next day. In mid-afternoon, as we came off the New Jersey Turnpike at Hightstown, a huge black mushroom cloud came boiling up out of the west and spread swiftly across the sky until it closed over us like a smothering tent. A pale lurid streak glimmered on the eastern horizon for a few minutes, then that, too, succumbed to the opaque pall. The afternoon turned into night, and we were buffeted by a barrage of rain, sleet, and snow. Even the heavens, it seemed, were scowling an omen.

7

THE VIRGINIA TRIP HAD BEEN, PSYCHOLOGICALLY, AN unmitigated disaster. The emotional damage to my wife was deep, long-lasting, irreversible. First there had been the depressing George Washington University Hospital experience in 1964—hopes raised and dashed. Then this. Julia was never to be the same again.

She had nerved herself to face the surgical ordeal she dreaded. She had gone to Virginia courageously, her old optimism supporting her, hoping to be cured of her heart problem, and to be home in three weeks. When the shattering letdown came, she could be optimistic no longer. A sense of doom and futility overwhelmed her.

All this was not as clear immediately as it became months and years later, but at least one fact was instantly obvious: the Virginia episode never should have happened. My wife should never have been sent down there under the impression that she was going to have surgery, when there had been no adequate communication between The Great Doctor and Dr. Dammann. This lack of communication, I was to find, is typical of the splintered American medical system. Swamped by patients, doctors operate on a rush-rush schedule; patients walk out the door of an office or hospital and that is it. They are out of one expert's hands, into another's. As

Senator Edward M. Kennedy has written, "Each of the specialists and institutions frequently assumes that his individual responsibility begins and ends when a person crosses his doorstep."

In my wife's case, The Great Doctor had evidently convinced himself that, because Dr. Bailey favored an operation, Dr. Dammann would come to the same conclusion. He had sent us off to Virginia on this assumption. Obviously he had made no attempt to check closely with Dr. Dammann, because he had not even been aware until we phoned him that the gremlins had made off with Julia's records and that Dr. Dammann had never seen them. From Dr. Dammann's strong reaction to Julia's weight problem, I can only conclude that, had there been any appropriate consultation, The Great Doctor would never have been under the impression that Julia was almost certain to have surgery.

The entire episode should have warned us that The Great Doctor, with all his board certifications, with all his sophisticated skills, was gravely deficient in one vital aspect of medicine—attention to detail. Ironically, he had devoted a lot of time and consideration to Julia's problems; he had weighed the overall picture carefully—and then he could not be bothered to make a phone call to check with Dr. Dammann before he sent us off on that wild-goose chase.

My daughter, who had worked for a time for a firm of orthopedic specialists in our area, was incensed by The Great Doctor's nonperformance and wanted her mother to change physicians. "You just don't *do* such things," she told Julia and me with biting emphasis. "Our doctors would *never* send a patient off for surgery without making sure that the surgeon had had a chance to examine all the records and thought surgery was advisable. You just don't send a patient off telling her she's going to have open-heart surgery without talking to the surgeon *after* he's had a chance to study all her records."

Barbara obtained the names of other cardiologists in our area and urged her mother to consult one of them. But Julia would not. The Great Doctor had, indeed, stabilized her longer and more successfully than anyone else; she had come to look upon him as her last hope, her savior.

It soon became obvious, however, how the Virginia fiasco had altered her attitude in other respects. The Virginia team had been impressed when they learned that Julia took long walks with our collie dog almost every morning. An early riser, she would walk the dog almost a mile to the end of our town. Then she would rest awhile and start back. By the time I woke, the pair of them would often be only two or three blocks from home. One of the Virginia specialists asked me if she really did this, and when I said she did indeed, he nodded. "That's good," he said. "It shows what she can do." The Virginia specialists were anxious for her to continue such walks; the exercise, they pointed out, was good for her heart.

But after we came back from Virginia—in the 5½ years that were left—Julia never once walked our collie, not even for half a block. When I would remind her that the doctors wanted her to walk, she would alibi that the weather was too cold or too windy; and when the weather was neither, when she had no excuse, a stubborn, almost mulish look would cross her face, and she would insist: "I can't. I'm not strong enough."

Nearly six years later, after Julia's death, I discussed this entire sequence with Dr. Ebert in New York Hospital. He prefaced his remarks by saying, "If your wife came in to us today in the same condition she was in in 1968, we would operate without a moment's hesitation." The science had advanced that much in those few short years; it was Julia's fate that the timing for her was all wrong.

When I described the change in her after Virginia, Dr. Ebert nodded in understanding. It meant that Julia had given up on herself. "She may have thought you or the doctors were holding something out on her, and she was worse than you were willing to tell her," he suggested.

"No," I told him, "I don't think it was that. I think it was just that she had been sent all the way down there to be operated on—and she had been rejected. After that, I think she considered herself a hopeless case and quit."

Dr. Ebert nodded again. "Yes," he said, "that would have been the reaction." And he added that the burden of carrying this sense of rejection and hopelessness around for almost six years, in addition to the depressive pressures of the previous eleven years, must have had a shattering psychological effect.

There is no doubt that it did, for Julia now developed psychosomatic tendencies. Whenever she caught a cold, she would become so emotionally overwrought that symptoms of weakness and collapse would persist for as long as a month, well after the cold itself had been conquered. New medications had to be tried: tranquilizers to keep her from emotionally climbing the walls; mood-elevating drugs (these did not seem to have much effect) to bring her out of the depths of depression. The sudden escalation of medication shows in the entries in a small ledger I kept to record cash medical expenditures. Prior to the Virginia trip, year after year, the entries in this ledger would cover sometimes only a page, at most a page and a half, but in 1969 they covered four solid pages.

Another record that shows the change may be found in a diary that I kept. Beginning with the Virginia trip and continuing through 1969, I made regular, day-by-day entries; from these I have culled some significant excerpts. Typical is the sequence that began on November 10, 1969, when Julia came down with a cold.

I took her to The Great Doctor, and my entry reads: "He ordered some cough medicine for her. Found no congestion anywhere to worry about." But the next day, I noted: "Trouble. Mom's coughing her head off, feels like hell."

The problem got worse in this fashion:

> *Wednesday, November 12:* Sheer hell. She's dying, she says. Her eyes roll up in her head, and she throws it back to one side. Nobody, but nobody, knows how awful she feels. I'm to call the doctor tomorrow [Wednesday is doctors' day off in our area] to see what he can do. . . .
>
> *Thursday, November 13:* Doc ordered some more medicine for her, but she's no better in either mind or body. Doesn't think he knows what ails her—doesn't think *anybody* knows what ails her, how awful she feels. She's just *dying,* and *she* knows it.

This pattern continued for days until November 18, when Julia got up, got dressed, ate a good dinner for the first time, and "seemed better." But the next day she was again in a state of physical and emotional collapse. On November 24, The Great Doctor came to the house, examined Julia, could find no physical reason for her behaving as she was, and concluded she was working herself into a "state" and causing a lot of her own trouble. I noted, "He told her to stop 'acting like a child.'"

Temporarily, she seemed stronger, but in a couple of days she was in an emotional state again. She wracked herself coughing, yet she had no mucus to bring up. I took her to The Great Doctor on Monday, December 1. He examined her, found some slight traces of bronchial asthma, prescribed new medicine, and ordered us to come back in a week. My account of that second consultation follows.

> Julia's cold goes on and on. We saw the doctor at 7:30 P.M. He found her bronchial congestion nearly gone and talked to her for a long time about getting herself into such an emotional state when she is ill. She was biting her lips and nearly crying through it all. She cries at the drop of a hat—and especially at the thought of Christmas coming up.

Nobody ever reveled in Christmas more than Julia. With her warm heart, this was for her the greatest season of the year. She would begin baking up a storm ten days ahead of time, filling the house with the delicious aroma of cookies and crullers and other good things to eat; and her joy in buying presents, her delight in anticipating the delight of others in receiving them, cast a special loving glow over the entire holiday season. Whether it was the idea of not wanting to miss all this, or whether The Great Doctor's tough talk penetrated on this occasion, I do not know, but the results were immediately apparent. After that December 8 conference, Julia turned off her illness as one might turn off a water spigot, and plunged into happy preparations for Christmas. The upturn was to last her barely through the holidays.

8

CHRONIC ILLNESS SEEMS AT TIMES TO TRIGGER AN unrelieved series of disasters, a chain of successive blows, one following upon another, until the victim begins to feel pursued by a malignant fate that will prevent anything from ever coming out right again. In Julia's case, there was no respite from the shocks. The psychologically damaging hospital experiences of 1964 and 1968 were followed by what to her was a major physical disaster in the winter of 1970.

Ironically, her own great overweening mother's love was indirectly responsible for the event that was to deprive her of the one avocation in which she had found pleasure and solace.

No woman ever worshiped children more than Julia. To me, children at times can be obstreperous little devils; she saw them all, indiscriminately, as God's little angels. This mother's love of hers embraced all children, not just her own but anybody's; and so, naturally, she became almost dotty where her own grandchildren were concerned. She smothered them with uncritical affection, and they adored her.

Barbara's boys, like all small children, picked up colds in nursery school or from neighborhood playmates.

Prudence dictated that Julia should stay away from them at such times, but she adored them so much she always managed to convince herself they were germ-free before they actually were. As a consequence, she contracted a succession of colds and was confined to the house for most of January and February of 1970. And then, in early March, just when she seemed to be recovering, came the worst.

March 5 was a balmy, springlike day, and I took Julia out for a short ride, thinking the air and the change from weeks of confinement would do her good. On our way home, she wanted to stop at Barbara's to see her grandchildren. I demurred because the children had had colds again, but Julia was insistent; she was certain it would be all right. It wasn't. Two days later, she was once more ill, and this time it was serious.

She developed a bad case of bronchitis. The Great Doctor had gone to Florida for a short vacation, and the cardiologist who was substituting for him examined my wife, became alarmed at the congestion that he found, and ordered her into the hospital. Medicated oxygen was administered to break up the hard mucus that had formed in her bronchial passages.

This time she was in the hospital for seventeen days. Several days after she was admitted, The Great Doctor returned from Florida and took over supervision of her case. He was disturbed by what he found. As I noted in my diary, on March 19:

> He says her heart has been strained, and he'll keep her in the hospital for another week. But then a decision will have to be made about how long we can let this go on. He'll talk to Dammann in Virginia about an operation if she

49

gets her strength back in six months or so. Problem is, he says, that if this goes on you reach a point at which nothing can be done. It's not a happy prospect.

Julia was having a bad time in the hospital. As was the case now whenever she was ill, she refused to eat; no matter what the food, she turned from it in revulsion and sent her dinner plate back virtually untouched. The Great Doctor would later comment that he had never realized before how little she could eat and still not lose weight. It was a kind of hunger strike that symbolized her deep depression and discouragement, and soon she had even more cause to be depressed.

One morning, when she started to say something, her voice suddenly went peculiar. Whenever she tried to speak, she squeaked. Her inability to control the pitch of her voice unnerved her and made her wonder what was happening to her. A throat specialist was called in to examine her. His verdict: the new strain on her heart had resulted in damage to a vocal cord.

The Great Doctor later diagrammed for me what had happened. He explained that a nerve runs alongside the vocal cord, then loops down around the aorta on the left side of the heart and runs along the side of the lung. Julia's heart had been so strained during this last illness that there had been a new, slight enlargement of the left side; this bulge had pinched the nerve, and the nerve in spasmodic reaction had kicked against the vocal cord, damaging it irreparably.

No debility could have been worse for Julia's state of mind. Music had been one of the great joys of her life. From the time she was a girl in high school, she had sung in church choirs; and, in recent years, despite her heart condition, she had derived some of her greatest pleasure from singing in her own Presbyterian choir in winter and the large Ocean Grove Auditorium choir during the summer. Now, her voice ruined, even this last pleasure was going to be denied her.

Both The Great Doctor and I recognized the damage this would do. Some people who have seen him in daily action have since described him to me as so blinded by his own ego as to lack any warmth and compassion. I can only say that he certainly didn't act this way with us. After he had explained what had happened, he said with a kind of groan, "Oh, God, Fred, we didn't need this one."

He fiddled, looking at the diagram he had drawn for me, obviously postponing the inevitable. Then he heaved a huge sigh and said: "I wish I didn't have to do it, but there's no help for it. Let's go in and see Julia." His manner was that of a man who knew he was going to have to pass a virtual death sentence and who hated his role.

When he repeated for Julia the explanation he had just given me, she got the implications immediately. "Is there any chance it will get any better?" she asked.

"I'm afraid not, Julia," he told her.

"Then that means I can never sing in the choir again?"

"I'm afraid so, Julia," he told her.

Then she cried.

I brought her home the next day, March 28. While I was waiting for her to get ready, one of the nurses on the floor spoke to me.

"Can't somebody in the family do something for her?" she asked. "Can't you take her out for rides or get her out to see her grandchildren?"

The well-meant suggestion rubbed me wrong because these were the very things I had been doing, and I snapped at the nurse more sharply than I intended:

"That's the reason she's in here now. Every cold she's had this year she's picked up from the children."

The nurse shook her head. "All I know is that something ought to be done," she said. "I've never seen anyone so depressed."

She was, of course, right about the problem. However, it was one thing to know the problem and another to find some way of coping with it. An operation, if successful, might have restored my wife to a measure of health and relieved the psychological pressures; but The Great Doctor reported that he had conferred with Dr. Dammann and that Dammann was unalterably opposed to an operation.

"So we'll just have to go along as before," The Great Doctor said.

It was not a prospect to alleviate the deepening sense of doom that was ruining the spirits of my wife.

"I guess I'm a pretty hopeless case," she said.

9

We now entered a new phase in which Julia would collapse at times for no apparent reason. I had become accustomed to the debilitating effects a cold or illness of any kind had upon her, but this was different. There seemed to be no logical cause for the new, strange symptoms that would leave her prostrated. Was her heart valve weakening? Were we nearing that dreaded time when her heart would become so bad she would be a helpless, bedridden invalid unless—always that fearful question and doubt—a heart operation could save her?

In examining her, The Great Doctor could find no apparent physical change to account for her condition; and he finally decided in late January, 1972, to put her in the hospital for another heart catheterization to determine with precision what her damaged mitral valve was doing.

The local hospital had developed its own cardiology team, and it was no longer necessary to go into New York for such a procedure. The catheterization was performed smoothly and efficiently, and Julia was impressed by the competence of the examiners. Nevertheless, it was the same nerve-wracking, grueling operation: her arm where the catheter had been inserted, and where there had been some initial difficulty working it through the scar tissue caused by the previous test, was a battered black and blue; and she was thoroughly exhausted.

The results were far better than we had anticipated. The new catheterization showed that Julia's heart valve was in approximately the same condition as it had been five years previous; there had been no further deterioration, and so there was no need to rush into an operation. "What a surprise and relief!" I noted in my diary.

Essentially, however, Julia was left in limbo. She might be momentarily relieved by the knowledge that she was no worse, but at the same time she was left with no hope of getting any better. She still suffered from depression; she still had to drag through the days.

In the third week of March she suffered another of those mysterious physical letdowns that had made us fear earlier that her heart was failing. She collapsed on the couch in our living room, her head wobbling as if it might fall off at any moment, convinced she was going to die and telling me I would be better off if she did. In alarm, I made a special appointment for her with The Great Doctor, and on March 23 he gave Julia a thorough examination.

Again he could find no physical change to account for her condition: heart, chest, and lungs were all clear. There was no infection of any kind. He explained to us that Julia was so delicately balanced medically that she had no leeway, no real reserve of strength. And her deep depression sapped what strength she did have. I noted at the time: "This kind of depression comes from her kind of heart ailment, he said, and the depression makes the chronic fatigue that is there all the time that much worse —and this leads to new depression, and so on in a vicious circle."

Hunting for some way to combat this emotional drag, The Great Doctor encouraged Julia to undertake part-time volunteer work with the Monmouth County Heart Association. She began going into the office three mornings a week, working from 9 A.M. until noontime, and she found to her surprise that, by using an electric typewriter, she could address envelopes and prepare office records. As was typical of her with anything she undertook, she was soon pushing herself to get out ever more work. Now I had to caution her to slow down, to rest and pace herself, arguing that there was no need to finish a long mailing list in one morning; the rest of it could wait until next time. "Don't exhaust yourself," I'd tell her. "I wanted to get it finished," she'd answer.

There was no doubt that the volunteer work was good therapy for her. It got her out of the house; she formed new friendships, developed new interests; her mind was diverted from its sick preoccupation with her condition.

The Great Doctor, who had devised this psychological prop for her, continued to study her basic physical problem with the greatest care. When he went to national cardiologists' conventions, he took her records with him and conferred with some of the nation's leading specialists, seeking their advice about what should be done. After one convention in California, he told us he had been fortunate enough to get two preeminent men in the field to examine Julia's case in detail. Their advice was the same that he had received from others: "Leave it alone as long as she is as well as she is."

During these years The Great Doctor had been growing in stature in medical circles, developing a reputation that extended well beyond our local area. Interns from one of the largest and best hospitals in the East, Hahnemann in Philadelphia, came to the shore to train under him, and several of them became residents on his hospital staff. When such acolytes were following him around, Julia sometimes became a prize exhibit on whom he had them test their skills. I recall one occasion when The Great Doctor telephoned and asked Julia whether she would mind making a special trip into his office on a day when she did not have an appointment: he wanted to see how one of his students would perform in diagnosing her condition. Understandably, Julia got the feeling that she was a special patient, a circumstance that made the final oversight and neglect of basic detail that cost her her life something that one could not have imagined except in wildest fantasy.

There were, perhaps, faint warning signs that we should have heeded, but at the time they seemed such minor straws in the wind that it would have been silly to attach too much importance to them. As The Great Doctor became more involved in the work and administration of the hospital, he became more rushed and harried in handling his ever-increasing load of office patients. On occasion, some hospital snafu would delay him half or three-quarters of an hour in getting back to his office for his afternoon schedule of appointments; and then it was a case of rush-rush to catch up.

I recall an incident that seemed minor at the time, but that was perhaps not without its significance. On one of The Great Doctor's harried afternoons, Julia had an appointment for an examination, and the drugstore had asked me to get a renewal of her digoxin prescription. The Great Doctor snatched a pad, murmuring "twenty-five milligrams" to himself, and began to write out the prescription.

"No, that's not right," I told him. "She's taking fifty milligrams a day."

He paused. "Oh, is she?" he asked. He had forgotten the proper dosage, that first and most significant change he had made in her medical treatment. "Oh, well," he said, handing me the prescription he had finished, "have her take the twenty-five milligrams twice a day."

There was at least one other major change in The Great Doctor's handling of patients. When we had first gone to him, he had been willing to make house calls when Julia became ill; but he did that no longer. Now, when a crisis arose, he practiced medicine by telephone. I would describe Julia's symptoms to his office nurse or to the great man himself; and he would have his nurse phone a prescription for an antibiotic, a tranquilizer, or whatever he deduced the symptoms required. Since nearly all overworked doctors in our area were practicing medicine in this way, we became accustomed to the remote-control method of caring for patients. And so later, when we should have objected most strongly, we had become too conditioned to complain.

In this fashion the months passed, and Julia, despite her ups and downs, seemed at times to feel much better. The year 1973 was an especially good time for us—the last of the good times, as it turned out. Julia was happy in her job at the heart association, and she seemed to have found some secret reservoir of strength. The summer that year was especially hot and muggy along the Jersey shore, with temperatures in the high nineties late in June. This is normally bad weather for heart patients. But Julia, paradoxically, seemed to thrive on it and feel better than she had in years.

I remember one summer afternoon, hot and humid inland, when we went down to the oceanfront at a dead-end street in Deal. There, above the rock bulkhead, winter storms had hurled some massive pilings, now half-buried in the sand with wiry dune grass sprouting around them. We went down to an isolated little niche above the bulkhead below the end of the street. Julia sat down and leaned her back against one of the pilings, and I stretched out in the sand with my head in her lap. The sun shone hot and warm upon us; a gentle southeast breeze, laden with the tang of salt spray and seaweed, swept in off the ocean, cool and soothing; and we spent a quiet hour there, at peace with the world.

Julia was so amazed at how well she felt that she asked me, "Do you think my heart could be curing itself?"

I knew it wasn't possible, but I didn't want to say that. I could only tell her, "I hope so."

10

THE COLLAPSE CAME WITH SHOCKING SUDDENNESS, ES-pecially since it followed so closely that brief burst of well-being. With the onset of colder weather and the pro-liferation of viruses, Julia began her customary annual struggle with those minor illnesses that sapped her strength. But this time she must have felt within herself a tragic difference: she became obsessed with a presenti-ment that she had not long to live.

Early in the new year, she discussed with a long-time friend from her choir-singing days the music she wanted played at her funeral. She hoped the choir would sing the "Hallelujah Chorus" from *The Messiah* by Handel. She impressed upon me that she wanted no viewing; she wanted a closed casket so no one could look at her after she was dead. Get it over with as quickly as possible, she said.

It was macabre, and it made me frantic. I upbraided her for dwelling on such morbid thoughts; I tried to shut off such discussions, tried to get her mind to focus on other things. I had little success. Looking back afterward, I became convinced that, through some extrasensory per-ception I could not understand, she *knew*; but at the time I rebelled at the very thought of the possibility of her death.

Despite my rebelliousness, it was clear to me that Julia was failing. Her complexion still retained that rosy glow usually indicative of good health, so much so that even long-time neighbors and many of our friends thought that she was ten years younger than she actually was. Those of us who were close to her, however, could sense the physical letdown. On many occasions, she could no longer put in three hours' work at the heart association; she would be exhausted after a couple of hours and would telephone me to come and pick her up.

Sometimes she would stop to visit a good friend of hers, Mrs. Margaret Edelson, the widow of a doctor who had been one of the best in our area, and Margaret told me afterward: "You could see that she was failing badly in the last six months. Why, sometimes when she came to see me, she could just about crawl through that door before she collapsed in a chair."

Her dragging walk, her obvious physical slump, conveyed their message to The Great Doctor when she visited his office for her regular examinations. There seemed to be no serious alteration in her observable physical condition: there was no buildup of fluid around her heart, and she remained stabilized as she had been for years. But The Great Doctor could tell by keen observation that some subtle, hidden changes must be taking place in the functioning of the mitral valve, and he downgraded her several notches on a scale he used to indicate the functional well-being of heart patients.

In late spring he informed us that Dr. Ebert, the distinguished chief of the Department of Surgery at New York–Cornell, was coming down to the shore to review a number of critical heart cases with a panel of local cardiologists. The Great Doctor said that he would like Dr.

Ebert to examine Julia personally before the panel met. Could I bring her into his office in the early morning?

We kept the appointment, of course; but, again, it was one of those rush-rush affairs. Dr. Ebert had been delayed in leaving the city, had been tied up in traffic on the New Jersey Turnpike; and, by the time he arrived, the other cardiologists were already waiting for him in the hospital. He had only a few minutes to devote to Julia, but he studied her heart X rays and read the report of her 1972 catheterization with great care. Then he and The Great Doctor went into the inner examining room, where my wife was waiting.

They came out in a few minutes and rushed off to their meeting. "There's no time now, but I'll explain everything to you at Julia's next appointment," The Great Doctor told me as they departed.

My wife came out of the examining room and said, low-voiced, "He says I have to have it."

Medical science had made such strides in the six years since our trip to Virginia that the hazards of such an operation had been greatly reduced. Surgical techniques were now much improved over the methods in use then; and, as Dr. Dammann had predicted, the new heart valves were functioning with much greater efficiency.

"Dr. Ebert says I won't have nearly as good a chance a year from now," my wife told me, "but if I'm operated on now, I should have a ninety percent chance of coming through."

Dr. Ebert's personality and his optimistic assessment of my wife's chances gave Julia an enormous psychological lift. She had an uncanny ability to evaluate people accurately on first acquaintance. Call it feminine intuition or whatever you will; I only know that, whatever it was, her instinct was nearly infallible. Julia herself could never explain how she arrived at such judgments; she just *knew*, and events almost invariably demonstrated that she was right. So now her reaction to Dr. Ebert was not to be discounted. "He has the kindest eyes I've ever seen on a man," she told me. She liked him and put complete trust in him on the spot.

So remarkable was the effect that Dr. Ebert had on her that the months-long presentiment of impending doom seemed lifted from her. Her decision to take Dr. Ebert's advice and have the operation as soon as possible was made by the time we left The Great Doctor's office that spring morning; and she seemed to feel a great surge of relief that the uncertainty was over, the decision made. In highest spirits, she went off to tell a couple of close friends of thirty-five years' standing that she was going to have her operation; and she was further encouraged when their son, himself an excellent surgeon, rejoiced that she was going to have it done at New York–Cornell. This, he assured her, was one of the nation's greatest hospitals, and there, if anywhere, she should have every chance of coming through the surgery and feeling better than she had in years.

Buoyed by this reassurance, she amazed everyone by the cheerfulness, almost the eagerness, with which she faced the surgical ordeal whose prospect had haunted us and shadowed our lives for seventeen years. Recalling her attitude afterward, one of the policemen in our town, a long-time friend of both of us, shook his head in amazement. "I couldn't get over it," he said. "You might think she was going off to a tea party. If that had been me, I would have been terrified and you would have had to drag me kicking and screaming, but she seemed to face it as if it was nothing."

We had two weeks to wait before the appointment at which The Great Doctor was to "explain everything" to us, a delay that might have been expected to erode my wife's high spirits; but, to all appearances, it did not. She remained cheerful and optimistic.

This ebullient mood was all but destroyed by the events of June 6. That was the day of our afternoon appointment with The Great Doctor, and we were ushered into his inner office where we waited—and waited. The Great Doctor had been delayed by hospital problems, and he was an hour late in getting back to his office. There we were waiting for him; three other patients whose appointment times had come and gone were in the outer office, and more were due to arrive at any moment.

Tense and harried, The Great Doctor was in a tearing hurry to catch up. He went into the examining room, whipped out his stethoscope, and began to listen to Julia's heart. She looked at me, a faint smile on her face, as she said to him, "When am I going to have my heart operation?"

"Oh," he said, jocularly, "are you going to have a heart operation? I didn't know that."

She told him that she had decided to take Dr. Ebert's advice, and he summoned his nurse and told her to telephone Dr. Ebert's office and ask his assistants to get in touch with us to make the necessary arrangements. Then, obviously feeling the pressure of the backlog of waiting patients, he prepared to get rid of us.

While my wife was dressing, I asked him whether Dr. Ebert himself would perform the operation, an important consideration with her. He snapped at me as if I had asked something idiotic: "Of course! If he didn't Bill Gay would do it, and he's just as good. But she's Ebert's patient; of course he'll do it."

I asked him how long she might be in the hospital, and he said probably from ten to fourteen days. I expressed some surprise, because we had been prepared for a three-week hospitalization in Virginia only six years before. He explained that the mitral-valve operation was one in which such enormous strides had been made that patients rarely stayed more than two weeks now.

My wife joined us and, very tentatively, asked him a question. She had been wondering, I knew, about how soon she might be able to get back to her job at the heart association, being afraid that, if she were away too long, it might be necessary to get someone else to do her work. And so she asked how long it might take her to recuperate.

"How do I know? What am I? God?" he snapped, slapping his pen against her records in disgust.

That about ended the interview in which he had promised to discuss "everything" with me and my wife. As we left his office and walked down the hall, Julia was upset, unnerved, the high spirits that had sustained her dashed at one stroke.

"He told us he was going to tell us 'everything,' " she said, "and he didn't tell us anything. I don't think he cares. I don't think I'll have the operation."

I know that if I had agreed with her at that point, she would have abandoned the whole project—and she would, in all probability, have had at least a few more years of life. But I was convinced that her condition had deteriorated to the point where the operation that we both had dreaded for so long represented her one chance for a longer and better life. And so (how I would regret this later!) I argued with her and made excuses for The Great Doctor. I pointed out that he had been so swamped with hospital work and his sea of patients that he just hadn't been able to take the time with us that he had intended. But this, I said, didn't mean he didn't care. And I reasoned that she had gone too far now to back out, that she should still take Dr. Ebert's advice because she wouldn't have as good a chance later as she had now.

She agreed with this in the end; but the disillusioning encounter with the snappish Great Doctor continued to bother her and sapped some of her confidence. She began to ask me for the first time, a bit doubtfully, "Do you think he's a *really good* doctor?"

I told her, heaven help me, that I thought he was; he had such stature in our area that, at mention of his name, people would say, "Oh, he's good." I pointed out that he had worked hard in trying to judge her case, conferring with some of the top specialists in the profession, and that he had kept her system in balance all these years as no one else had been able to do before. I passed over in my mind other disturbing indications to which, I know now in retrospect, I should have given more consideration.

But I felt confident at this point—and I think that Julia to a great extent did too—that all would turn out well. Julia's operation would be performed by Dr. Ebert, the chief of the Department of Surgery at New York–Cornell, one of the truly great hospitals. You couldn't do any better than that. And when Julia came home, she would be in the care of The Great Doctor, the chief of the Department of Medicine in the largest and probably the best hospital in our area. You couldn't do better than that. How could anything go wrong?

11

THE DATE WAS SET. JULIA WAS TO GO INTO THE HOSPITAL on June 26 and have her operation on June 28. It was a tight schedule, and the events were supposed to run like clockwork; but, from the beginning, the clock did not tick smoothly. Julia's story now became the story of countless others, illustrative of the consequences of an overburdened, chaotic medical system.

June 26 was a nerve-wracking day, a time of such tension that it could not help but have an adverse effect on my wife. Her admission to the hospital had been scheduled for two weeks—but there were no beds.

We had been told that the hospital would call us when it was ready to receive my wife, but noontime came and there was no word. I telephoned Dr. Ebert's office, and his secretary told me that the admissions staff expected some afternoon discharges; they would notify us when they had found a bed.

Mid-afternoon came; still no word. I telephoned again since my wife was biting her nails and muttering that she might call the whole thing off. There was still not a bed to be had, Dr. Ebert's secretary said; but she added that Dr. Ebert had "read the riot act" to the admissions people, telling them they just *had* to come up with a bed because he had an operation to perform that had been scheduled for two weeks. All we could do was wait some more; they would let us know.

It was five o'clock in the afternoon before the call came through; a bed had been found at last. I could bring my wife to the hospital now.

Julia's nerves were almost in tatters by this time. She had begun the day looking remarkably well. At a friend's house in the morning, a much younger woman who, as a girl in high school, had known my wife years before, commented in amazement that she didn't look much different than she had in those younger and healthier days. Another friend who saw us that morning, and who had no idea she was facing heart surgery, reacted with surprise and shock when I told him the next day that she was in the hospital. "Oh, God, no!" he said; "I can't believe it. She looked so beautiful, *so beautiful,* when you were in here yesterday morning."

She had nerved herself up for the day; she was, I suppose, keyed up, and this no doubt helped to enhance her appearance. But by late afternoon, after hours of nerve-frazzling uncertainty, she had lost much of her bloom and bounce.

We had an hour-and-a-half drive up the Garden State Parkway, along the New Jersey Turnpike to the Lincoln Tunnel, and through the congestion of cross-town, rush-hour traffic before we could get up the East Side to the hospital at Sixty-eighth Street and York Avenue. It was a drive I will never forget.

Massive dark clouds closed in low over the turnpike, and the noisome petrochemical concentrations around the Amboys were spewing flame and smoke into the pall like something out of Dante's inferno. It had been bright daylight when we left home, but the black cloud cover blotted out the sun and imposed a nighttime gloom, shot through with the lurid industrial spoutings. We had the car windows closed and the air conditioning on; but the reek of the oil refineries that lined the road penetrated every tiny aperture and made my wife gag. It was a scene fit for a canvas depicting the landscape of hell.

Julia's mind turned to many things on that drive. I had just finished a book on which I had been working the whole first half of the year, but she hadn't read the manuscript because, she said, she thought she would get a greater thrill out of reading the published work. Had she been right to wait? she wondered now. I told her I could understand how she felt about waiting for the book itself; no, I didn't think she had been wrong. Later, thinking back, I could see that her remark was open to morbid interpretation. Was she beginning to doubt she would live to read it?

At another point on that dreary drive, she asked me, "You wouldn't miss me too much if I wasn't here, would you?"

I thought she should have known after all our years together how much I would miss her, and the question angered me. "Oh, for Christ's sake, dear," I told her, "I'd be lost and lonely and miserable without you."

"Well, perhaps for a little while," she said. "But you'd soon get over it. You'd have the dog and your work."

"Oh, for Christ's sake!" I exclaimed in disgust. I couldn't stand this kind of talk. The dog and my work, indeed! Later, I would become convinced that she was worrying about me, trying to convince herself that, even if the worst happened, I would be all right and wouldn't suffer too much.

The same concern showed in another remark she made. "Don't try to come and see me every day," she said. "It will be too much for you. There isn't any use your coming in tomorrow because they'll probably have me busy undergoing tests all day and you wouldn't have much chance to see me anyway."

Since this seemed logical, I said, to my infinite later regret, "All right."

"And there really isn't any sense in your coming in for the operation," she pursued. "There's nothing you can do, and I'll be out of it: I wouldn't even know whether you were there or not."

At this, I balked. "Listen," I told her, "Barbara and I are going to be there, no matter what. I want you to know when you go into that operating room that we're both there, rooting for you, and that we're going to stay until we can be certain you're all right."

It was a little after six-thirty by the time we reached the hospital; and after I had made the arrangements for her admittance, I left her there and drove back home. As we had agreed, I did not go into the hospital the next day, but by mid-afternoon I had cause to wish I had.

Julia telephoned me in a panic. A nurse had just briefed her fully on the gory anatomical details of the operation she was to undergo the next morning. This was a development I had not anticipated. I had reasoned that there was no point in unnerving her with such detailed information; full knowledge about the shocking, frightening procedure could only destroy her confidence instead of helping her to survive the ordeal she faced.

"Do you know what they are *going to do to me?*" she wailed to me now on the phone.

"Yes, dear, I know," I told her. "It's something that can't be helped, but remember they do this kind of an operation now almost as successfully as a simple appendectomy. You'll be all right."

Nothing reassured her; she sounded as if she were going to pieces—and there I was stuck at home some fifty miles away from her. When she hung up, I began cursing, blaming myself for being all kinds of a fool in not being with her to sustain and comfort her. After I had kicked the chair and scared the dog and ranted to my son and daughter, who had just come into the house, I calmed down enough to think about doing something to rectify the situation. And I telephoned The Great Doctor.

"I have just talked to Julia," he told me. "I think I calmed her down, and she'll be all right."

Why, in God's name, I asked, had it been necessary to scare the daylights out of her?

"Look, Fred," he said, "the hospitals in New York have to do this to protect themselves against malpractice suits. If they don't and something goes wrong, then the family says, 'Poor old Papa Joe would *never* have had the operation if he had known, and you killed him.' And then they sue. The hospitals just can't leave themselves open to this kind of charge; they have to make certain the patient knows everything in advance; and, unfortunately, we've had a couple of cases where patients who really needed the operation have refused to have it and have practically run screaming out of the hospitals when this was explained to them."

It was my first awareness of an issue that was to mushroom into a medical crisis as malpractice-suit losses led some insurance companies to double their premium demands and compelled others to stop writing policies. After The Great Doctor's explanation, I could understand that the hospital had had to brief my wife in detail, regardless of the psychological damage; but afterward, looking back, I would become convinced that the whole business should have been handled differently. Shouldn't The Great Doctor, knowing that such an explanation was inevitable, have given my wife the details himself at that last conference at which he had been going to tell her "everything"? Certainly, if she had to know, it would have been better then, with me there to lend her whatever support I could; she should not have been alone in a distant hospital, far from anyone she knew, when this was sprung on her. If she had to be terrified by too-specific knowledge, better it should be done before her decision to have the operation became almost irrevocable; better she should face the matter with her eyes open than go in blind and be scared almost out of her wits on the verge of the operating table.

Later, too, like the relatives of other heart patients, I would question what seems a dual system of ethics. Granted the need of the hospital staff to protect themselves on the malpractice front, their concern seemed largely for themselves, not for the psychological welfare of their patient. All major surgery is a shock to the system; "postoperative depression" is a common term applied to a recognized phenomenon. The aftereffects are especially severe in open-heart surgery; the psychological damage is often destructive, sometimes irreparable. Yet, as Julia's case demonstrates, almost no effort is made to prepare the patient and the patient's family for the onset of such problems; and without preparatory effort, the problems become magnified, mysterious, overwhelming.

"They tell you nothing that will help you to deal with things after the operation." This was a complaint that, in the months ahead, I was to hear again and again. It was certainly true in our case. The whole emphasis was on the surgery, on the success of the surgical procedure; that hurdle passed, there were supposed to be no serious problems. So we were led to believe.

12

No heart surgery could have gone more smoothly; no patient could have come through it better; no prognosis could have been more favorable. The day after Julia's operation, tubes were being removed from her body; by Sunday, after less than forty-eight hours in intensive care, she was well enough to be moved to a semiprivate room on the floor. "But it's the weekend," the resident in charge told me, "so we'll keep her in intensive care until Monday morning, though actually she's well enough to be moved now."

When I saw her Monday, she looked remarkably well, considering what she had endured. The usual long ugly scar ran down the center of her chest; her whole rib cage was hideously black and blue from the violence done to it in surgery; there were deep black-and-blue bruises on her arms. But her facial color was remarkably good. She breathed without difficulty, and she talked to me with perfect coherence.

Dr. Ebert was making his rounds, and I followed him out into the hall to inquire about my wife's condition. "Oh, she's doing fine," he assured me. "She's going to be all right. Look at her now [pointing]; she's already sitting up."

She was, indeed. She was sitting erect, swinging her

legs over the side of the bed, looking out her window at boats going up and down the East River.

It was beautiful; it was marvelous. The euphoria we had felt Friday afternoon when Julia had come through the operation so well seemed to have been fully justified. We soared again.

Yet there were subtle indications of potential trouble. One of the nurses had told me on Sunday: "She's doing fine. But we have one problem; she's not eating. That doesn't disturb us—yet."

That "yet" disturbed me. I was with Julia when her noon meal was brought in; she looked at it and made a face. "I can't eat it," she said. "It will make me sick."

I tried to coax her, cutting her meat and trying to feed it to her. She took a couple of tiny nibbles, one small spoonful of mashed potatoes, a couple of small pieces of fruit, and that was it. She wouldn't even drink her tea. "I can't," she said. "You drink it."

This attitude annoyed me as it had for years. "Look, dear," I told her, "you should be ecstatic that you have come through the operation so well, but you cannot get your strength back unless you make an effort. You've got to eat."

"I can't," she said. "I feel sick to my stomach." She was being stubborn again. Her mind was set.

There were things I didn't know, things that nobody bothered to tell me. I was so ecstatic at the way she had survived the long-dreaded operation that I thought she should be ecstatic, too. I had no idea that very few persons coming through this brutal surgery feel that way; that, on the contrary, the shock to the physical and nervous systems is so severe that many develop dangerous, even crippling, psychological blocks, and some even become paranoid. In view of what I later learned, Julia was not acting as badly as I thought at the time, but it was obvious, nevertheless, that she was being a difficult patient.

"The nurses have all been nice," she said to me, "except for one night nurse."

"What did she do?" I asked.

"She said to me, 'I don't have to take this shit.' "

"Well, what had you done to make her say that?"

A closed, mulish look came over my wife's face, the kind of look she got when she wasn't going to tell you something.

"Oh, I just asked her a question," she evaded.

"You must have done more than that," I said.

She didn't say anything more, but it was obvious to me that she must have been fussing up a storm to make a trained nurse react in that fashion.

After Julia took her noon pills, she began to drowse. She was being heavily sedated to help her bear the postoperative pain, especially excruciating after heart surgery. She murmured good-bye to me as she dropped off to sleep, and I left her, convinced that she was going to be all right.

The first shock came on Wednesday night. I had not gone in to see Julia on Tuesday, as we had agreed. Barbara and a friend, Linda Madden, had intended to see her Wednesday; but, at the last moment, Barbara's children required her at home, and she couldn't make the trip. The unfortunate consequence was that no one in the family had been to see Julia for two days, and she was upset.

I happened to stop at Margaret Edelson's on my way home from dinner that night, and Margaret came hurrying to the door to greet me. "I'm glad you're here," she said. "I've got Julia on the phone, and she says nobody has been to see her since her operation."

Shocked, wondering what was happening, I talked to

my wife. I reminded her that I had seen her on Monday, described the way we had talked together, tried to recall to her mind that I had been there when Dr. Ebert was making his rounds and that I had left only after her noontime sedatives began to take effect. Didn't she remember that I had sent her a bouquet of yellow rosebuds for her room? No, she had no recollection of any of it.

What had happened? I was appalled. I could not know—and no one had bothered to explain—that such lapses of memory and, indeed, even more serious mental impairments are commonplace in open-heart surgery cases. At the time, I ascribed my wife's memory lapse to the heavy sedation necessary to relieve postoperative pain, but I know now that something much more serious was involved.

When I saw Julia the next day, she still had no recollection of my Monday visit, and she was still not doing much to help herself. I continued to be disturbed by her refusal to eat. When I argued with her that she just *had* to eat something, she said she might like some ice cream, and so I went out and got her some. But after a couple of tentative spoonfuls, she rejected that, too.

The contrast with the Puerto Rican woman in the next bed annoyed me. Dr. Ebert later told me that she had had a much more serious heart condition than my wife; she had had two valves that needed to be replaced. But she was a determined lady. Whenever meals were brought in, she got up out of bed, sat down in a chair, and forced herself to eat everything. She must have felt as nauseous at times as my wife, for one day she vomited up her food, much to her embarrassment. Still, she persisted, and I argued with Julia that she should make a similar effort. But she would not.

This refusal to help herself was aggravating. Julia told me that one of the day nurses had snapped at her,

"You may have been a woman once, but you're like a child now." What had caused such an outburst? She wouldn't say, but the remark upset her greatly and she repeated it to Margaret Edelson and others. She was aggrieved, but not spurred to change her ways.

For the rest of that week, one or more of us in the family were with her every day. During these visits, certain subtle indications emerged to which, if we had known, we would have attached more importance. She began to remark, without making any particularly big issue of it, that she was seeing things that were not there: boats on the river, for example.

She was obviously hallucinating, but I put this down to the effect of the drugs she was being given. We had had an example of this only a couple of years previously. A close friend of ours had a serious operation, was placed on painkilling medications—and went almost out of his mind. Lying there in his hospital bed, he became convinced that he was driving an ambulance into New York and was crashing it right across the sidewalk and into the lobby of the *Daily News* on East Forty-second Street. Why this particular fantasy should have taken such vivid hold on his mind he never knew, but it was as real to him at the time as if it were actually happening. Hospital attendants had all they could do to keep him in bed and away from the wheel of that imaginary ambulance. Compared to such extreme reactions, Julia's hallucinations seemed relatively mild and harmless. But they were not, as we would ultimately learn.

Typical of the way she was acting was her conduct on Friday when Barbara and Linda visited her. It was now just a week after her operation. She was getting stronger all the time; but, instead of being encouraged, she exhibited her old tendency to exaggerate her condition in a play for sympathy. The girls were late getting into the city, and Julia told them truthfully she had been up and down and out in the hall looking for them a dozen times before they arrived. (Dr. Ebert would comment to me later about how remarkably ambulatory she had been.) But when Julia needed to go to the bathroom after Barbara and Linda came, she tottered along, protesting that she was too weak to walk unless she held on to someone's arm.

I discussed some of these difficulties with a young nurse on the floor. She smiled and said: "She's enjoying her illness, isn't she? Well, we get them like that."

How was she really doing? I asked. "Oh, she's doing fine," the nurse assured me. "She has her little crying spell every morning, but she gets over it. And she's really getting stronger all the time. She's going to be all right."

Then, on Sunday, nine days after her operation, there came another shock. I was having breakfast at a luncheonette where we often ate, when the telephone rang. It was Julia. She was in another panic, even more hysterical than the one on the day she was briefed on the gory anatomical details of the operation. Talking to her, I could not get any clue to what had unnerved her; worried and anxious, I jumped into the car and drove into the city.

I found it difficult to talk to her. She had that closed, half-sullen, evasive look that I had come to recognize as meaning she was determined not to tell me something I wanted to know. I could not fathom what had caused her sudden hysteria. She was still hallucinating. She seemed more disturbed by the persistent false images than she had been; but this did not seem to be enough to account for her extreme reaction.

When her afternoon pills began to take effect, I prepared to leave. I was across the room, my hand on the knob of the door, when she looked at me from her bed and said in a piteous voice: "I know I'm not going to make it. I know I'm going to die."

That premonition of imminent death that had so obsessed her earlier in the year had obviously taken possession of her again. I felt, I regret to say, furious with her. She had cried wolf so often, she had been "dying" with so many colds, that I had little patience with her now. I was convinced—and am still—that there was no reason for her to die; she had demonstrated amazing physical strength and stamina in standing the operation so well. This premonition of death, I reasoned, was just a mental aberration from which she would recover as she got stronger. I put no credence in it.

13

THE VERY NEXT DAY, AS I STEPPED OFF THE ELEVATOR
on the eleventh floor of the hospital, I encountered a
bouncy young nurse, a girl who seemed to revel in her
job as she swept up and down the halls, giving the impression of being everywhere at once. "Your wife is going
to be discharged any day now," she told me.

I was surprised, especially since this news came less
than twenty-four hours after my disturbing Sunday ses-
sion with Julia, and I guess my astonishment showed.
The nurse explained: "Well, we're not really doing anything for her anymore except giving her her medications,
and she can get those just as well at home."

The word had obviously gone out that all of the
patients in my wife's four-bed, so-called semiprivate room
were scheduled for quick release; later, while I sat with
Julia, another nurse came in, calling out: "Walking time.
You're all going to be out of here in a couple of days."

I talked to Dr. Ebert on Tuesday, and he said, yes,
my wife was to be released soon; she could come home at
almost any time I wished to come and get her. My daughter had suggested that it might be a good idea to hire
daytime nurses when Julia first came home, and I asked
Dr. Ebert if my wife would need any special care.

"Oh, no," he said, "she will be perfectly fine on her

own. She will need some help with meals, but that is all."

This did not concern me since, for years, I had been doing most of the cooking. I told Dr. Ebert that I would come and get Julia any time he said, and it was finally agreed that I should bring my wife home on Thursday, just thirteen days after her operation.

Since Barbara and I were going into New York to bring her back, my son drove over from his home in northern New Jersey to spend Wednesday afternoon and early evening with Julia. And so it happened that he was with her when a group of residents and interns came in, making their final check. Julia had appeared depressed and fretful, and before my son left so that the hospital team could examine her, he heard her tell them, "I feel as if I have bubbles in my head."

Later that night when he told me about the "bubbles," both he and I laughed. Julia's habit of exaggerating her ills had conditioned us to discount much that she said, and this remark seemed to us especially ridiculous. "Oh, Mother has bubbles in her head, has she?" I said.

When I told Barbara about the incident, her reaction was the same as ours. "Bubbles in her head?" she repeated after me in astonishment. "What next?"

We had no way of knowing that Julia, on this occasion, had not been fanciful. She had given the hospital team, as we would learn much too late, a very precise description of what she was actually feeling, and that phrase, "bubbles in my head," should have alerted trained personnel to the fact that a serious problem existed.

When Barbara and I reached the hospital the next day, Julia was ready and waiting for us. She was not fully dressed, but was in nightgown and slippers, with a long robe covering her. It was nearly lunchtime when we arrived, and the nurse suggested that Julia should try to eat something before we left. Barbara and I started to go down to the cafeteria to get our lunch; but Julia seemed unreasonably, almost irrationally, upset at the idea of our leaving her for a minute.

"You won't go without me, will you?" she asked worriedly.

"For heaven's sake, no, dear," I told her. "That's why we're here. We came to get you."

When we returned to her room, a nurse briefed us on the medications Julia was to be given at home. The nurse handed us a printed instruction sheet and went through the list with us, giving us an additional oral briefing on some of the drugs and how they were to be administered. One was Coumadin, the blood-thinning agent Julia had taken before the electric-shock treatment a decade before. It was given to heart-surgery patients to lessen the danger of clots forming around the new valve. The printed instructions said:

> Since this drug works by decreasing the clotting of the blood, it may cause bleeding. Report any bleeding to your doctor, for Coumadin may be having too strong an effect on you. [A footnote to this said: "Changed diet and activity may also have an effect on Coumadin."] You will have periodic protime blood tests to check its effect on the clotting of your blood and the dosage will be regulated accordingly.

("Protime" is a contraction for prothrombin time, a measure of the clotting time of blood. The clotting time of a patient on blood-thinning drugs is measured against that of normal blood to insure that the patient's blood is not thinned out too much.)

"Periodic," of course, means nothing. A week? Two weeks? A month? It was all so casual that my daughter, who was listening with me, could not recall afterward that we had received any additional briefing. But I remember the nurse's saying: "Your doctor will arrange for your protime blood count, probably about a week after you return home. If you have a cut and it does not stop bleeding, notify your doctor because it will indicate the blood is too thin. If a bruise appears under the skin, it will mean the same thing, and so you should notify your doctor."

There was, it seemed, nothing to worry about there, and the subject was passed over so quickly, so casually, that it did not even jog a ten-year-old memory buried in the back of my skull—a lapse that all too soon was to burden me with the worst feeling of guilt I have ever endured.

While we were being briefed, another nurse was going through the same routine with the Puerto Rican woman and her husband, sitting on the adjacent bed. The wife had been in the hospital a few days longer than Julia, but then she had had a much more serious operation. Despite this it was evident that she had recovered much better than my wife. She was fully dressed, and when the nurse asked her if she wanted a wheelchair to take her downstairs, she replied, almost with scorn, "No, I don't need it." And swept out of the room with rapid, confident strides.

Julia needed a wheelchair; and while we were waiting in the hall for one to be brought, Dr. Ebert came along and smiled down at her in his kindly, reassuring fashion.

"Don't worry," he told her. "You are going to be fine when you get home—just fine."

She gave him a wan, half-hopeful smile.

We got Julia in the car and headed home, jolting through crosstown streets and down to the Lincoln Tunnel, a ride that must have been uncomfortable for her, to say the least. The jolting started some minute bleeding from two round puncture wounds that had not completely healed at the base of her rib cage. But there was no murmur of complaint from Julia; she sat quietly in the bucket seat beside me, dozing occasionally and rousing only to complain about the hallucinating images that still boggled her mind.

She remarked at one point that she was seeing people who were not there; at another, that she seemed to be looking into a pirate's chest filled with treasure. "That's nice, Mother," Barbara told her. "Save some of it for us, will you?" Julia smiled faintly.

The first days at home went fairly well. I was preoccupied (too preoccupied, perhaps, but then this was the only problem that had been emphasized to me) with my wife's continued rejection of food. I thought that, on some occasions, I got a better meal into her than she had been eating in the hospital; but, at best, it was a hit-and-miss proposition. She was not helping herself as she might have. But then the medical profession wasn't helping either: immediately, disturbing gaps in communication became apparent.

For example: I telephoned The Great Doctor on Friday to let him know how well my wife had stood the trip home. He was surprised, and I was amazed at his surprise: he hadn't known that she had come home; he had thought she was still in the hospital. And he had to ask *me* what medications she was getting.

Again: the nurse who had briefed us at the hospital had said that the Public Health Service in our area had been notified and would be sending a visiting nurse to the house to check on my wife. We heard nothing; and, on Monday, the health service told us it had never been contacted.

As the days passed, the gradual improvement I had anticipated did not seem to be taking place. I had had a hospital bed brought in and set up in the living room to make Julia as comfortable as possible, and I had intended to sleep on the couch beside her. But in the middle of the first night, she wanted the couch because it was softer, and I went upstairs to my own bed. That night, tired probably from the trip home, she slept soundly; but, after that, the nights became restless horror times.

She could not sleep. The sleeping pill prescribed by the hospital seemed to help for only a couple of hours; then she would be awake, uncomfortable, complaining of pain in her chest. (Dr. Ebert would tell me later that such nighttime restlessness is characteristic of heart-surgery patients, but he seemed to feel, much to my surprise, that Julia had borne pain well. "She seemed to have much less pain than most patients," he said, something that I would not have believed from the way she was acting at home.)

I was up and down three or four times a night, giving her a pill for the pain when enough time had elapsed so that she could have one, or Valium, a tranquilizer, to settle her nerves when she seemed almost ready to climb the walls. The broken nights, the worry and concern, began to make one day merge into another in a gray fog. I was so tired that I began to lose my grasp, and some things that happened slipped through my mind as through a vacuum. The major shocks were so severe that I can remember every detail, but some of the lesser developments that led up to them are lost beyond recall.

We seemed to go from Sunday crisis to Sunday crisis. On the first Sunday Julia was home—it was her third day back and just a week after she had told me in the hospital that she knew she was not going to make it—she became utterly distraught. I cannot, try as I will, remember the specifics. She was still hallucinating, and the persistence of these false images, I believe, had begun to unravel her nerves and make her fear she was losing her mind. I have no recollection of any particularly horrible vision; it seemed to be the accumulation, the persistence of the hallucinations, that drove her over the brink.

Sunday, of course, is the worst time of the week to get in touch with a doctor. The Great Doctor was understandably not available, and calling his answering service elicited no response. We tried to seek other medical advice but without success.

That night and the early hours of Monday morning were an especially restless, harried time. I tried to help and comfort Julia, but nothing I could do seemed to have much effect. Toward morning, I fell into a kind of stupor in my bed upstairs; and when I awakened, she was on the telephone. She had apparently raised such a storm with the answering service that the operator had broken regulations and put her through to The Great Doctor at home.

What she tried to tell him, I do not know, for it was just at this point that I became aware of what was happening. As I walked to the head of the stairs, Julia put the phone back in its cradle and said in a hurt, anguished voice:

"He hung up on me."

14

WE HAD NOW CROSSED THE GREAT DIVIDE AND WERE ON the downslope to ultimate disaster, but I had no conception of the reality. Like many others in such cases, I could see what was happening and not understand any of it. Love blinds the mind, making it reject the thought of the death of the loved one; certainly, I thought, Julia was going to get better—she just *had* to get better. Coupled with this instinctive, subconscious blocking out of the image of death was a second deluding factor: that unquenchable euphoria, the end product of the widely accepted cult of the surgeon.

The operation had gone so well, and the operation, in our minds all those years we had dreaded it, had been everything. Julia's tragic experience, duplicated with only minor variations in detail by numerous others, would educate me in time to the truth: that the most critical period for heart-surgery patients comes after the operation. No other operative procedure causes such a host of critical problems—problems that simply did not exist before—and both hospitals and doctors, themselves wedded to the cult of the surgeon, all too frequently ignore the newly created potentials for disaster.

This lack of comprehension showed in the attitude

of The Great Doctor when we got in touch with him that Monday afternoon. He was impatient with Julia, whom he had not seen since she returned home, and he obviously considered that she was kicking up an emotional, irrational fuss. Past experiences with her had conditioned him, of course, to jump to such a conclusion. In his eyes, she was simply "acting up" and nothing more serious was involved.

"She should be ecstatic that she has come through the operation so well," he told my daughter over the telephone. "This mental attitude of hers is a crock of shit."

For an expert, he displayed an appalling lack of understanding of what, as I later learned, were not unusual psychological reactions for a heart-surgery patient. I, too, had thought in my simplemindedness that Julia should have been "ecstatic," but I was not supposed to be an expert.

The hallucinations that were the underlying cause of most of my wife's distress did not seem to concern The Great Doctor very much. He apparently ascribed them, as I had, to the painkilling drug Julia was being given. This was Darvon, which is taken by many patients without any disturbing side effects, but which produces bad reactions in others. The hospital instruction sheet we had been given suggested the substitution of the milder Tylenol for Darvon if a change was to be made, and The Great Doctor ordered the switch now.

Following his instructions, I stopped the Darvon and substituted Tylenol that Monday afternoon. Shockingly, all that happened was that Julia's hallucinations escalated into new and more horrifying forms.

About one-thirty A.M. Wednesday, she called me, highly agitated. "Did we go out last night?" she asked.

No, I said, of course not. "Are you sure?" she persisted. "I saw a horrible accident in which the kids were killed."

I told her that she must have been having a nightmare, but an hour later she called me again. "I'm too old to be pregnant, isn't that right?" she asked. I said that certainly was right. "But I feel as if I'm pregnant," she said, sounding baffled and worried.

Another hour, and she called again. She was seeing a whole crowd of evil, grinning, leering faces. They looked like monsters who had killed people, she said. By this time, she was convinced that she was going crazy—and I was, too.

Such crises always seem to come at the worst possible times, on a weekend or, as now, on Wednesday, the doctors' day off. I tried without success to reach The Great Doctor through his answering service. Next, I telephoned the wife of a long-time friend, a woman who knew The Great Doctor socially, who had worked for years as a medical secretary and knew all the girls in the answering service. "I called four times," she told me later. "I explained I was an old, old friend of Julie and that I was worried about her, and I asked them to get through to the doctor and have him call me. Knowing those girls, I'm sure he must have gotten the message, but I never got a call back." Neither did I.

I finally reached the heart specialist who was covering for The Great Doctor on this Wednesday. He asked me if Julia's trouble had begun in the hospital. I said it had. "Oh, I know what it is then," he told me. He explained that in rare cases there is the briefest gap when the heart-lung machine takes over bodily functions. The failure to synchronize perfectly the operation of the machine with the freezing of the heart means that the right mixture of blood and oxygen does not get to the brain instantly, and there is some resultant brain damage. "I had a patient out in Cleveland Clinic to whom this happened," the doctor said. "But the point is that the brain damage will heal itself as the surgical scar does. The important thing is to reassure your wife. Try to convince her that she is not going crazy, that this is a thing that sometimes happens and it will pass."

I couldn't get Dr. Ebert in New York Hospital, but his colleague Dr. Gay called me back and confirmed this diagnosis. I asked what I should do, explaining that our local expert had wanted to get my wife off Valium as much as possible because it is a depressant and she was already too depressed. Dr. Gay agreed with the reasoning, but added that, in the circumstances, I had no choice but to continue with the Valium. "If this keeps up," he suggested, "perhaps she ought to be brought back into the hospital and be given some psychological help."

What impressed me most about this was that Dr. Gay could take the trouble to call me back from New York, but I never heard again from our resident experts. The Great Doctor's office told me the next day that the cardiologist who had been covering for him had, indeed, gotten in touch with him at a meeting he was attending. But The Great Doctor himself never got around to calling, in effect ignoring the whole problem.

One tortures one's self afterward with all the second-guessing of hindsight. It was at this point, I am convinced, that I should really have raised some hell; that I should have yelled and raged and threatened, and even, if possible, have gone to the extent of calling in another doctor to check on my wife. Unfortunately, this is not my nature; I am not the arrogant, screaming type; and I had, I suppose, too great an inclination to understand and sympathize with the problems of an overworked, overburdened, harried medical system. I knew The Great Doctor, with his multiple responsibilities, was a hard-driven man; and, as I had done before, I made excuses for him that, in retrospect, I feel he didn't deserve.

There was another factor. Having struggled through Wednesday, the doctors' off day when nothing more could have been done, we plunged into a day of fast-moving developments—a day that, though we could not know it at the time, was accursed with a couple of near-misses, such fatal conspiracies of circumstance that one becomes almost convinced that Julia had been clair-voyant in her premonition of death and that the outcome had been predetermined by some overriding, malignant fate.

Of one thing I am now certain: belated explana-tions of the heart-lung-machine gap, reassurance that she was not losing her mind, had no effect. I had explained to Julia at once on Wednesday what the doctors had told me; I had urged her not to worry, to banish the idea that she was going crazy; and she had nodded to me in a kind of numb agreement. Only later did I discover that she must have concluded she was being given a snow job.

On Thursday morning, Linda Madden, my daugh-ter's young friend, called on my wife. They talked quietly for some time. Much later, I learned that Julia had told her, "I know that my heart is fixed and that I can get well physically, but if I'm going to be insane I don't want to live."

Much later, too, I learned that Linda, who had had some nurse's training and had served for a time in an intensive care unit in a Boston hospital, had been shocked by Julia's growing pallor and general appear-ance. She had seen this look too many times on patients about to die not to recognize it, she told my daughter, and she added, "If something isn't done, I don't give her more than about four days to live."

Barbara didn't tell me this until much later, not wanting to worry me; but then, after all, whose opinion do you take? That of a young woman who has had some brief experience in intensive care? Or that of The Great Doctor himself? For he rendered an entirely contrary and utterly emphatic opinion on this crucial day.

The final tangle that was to lead to tragedy began with The Great Doctor's arrangements for a blood test. There had been some vague mention of the necessity for such a test, but no specific time had been set until now. The Great Doctor set up this schedule: I was to bring my wife to the main entrance of the hospital before 2:00 P.M. the next day, Friday; there she would be directed to the lab. And at 3:30 P.M. I was to bring her to his office for examination.

The Public Health Service nurse, who made her second call on my wife on this same Thursday afternoon, was shocked by this arrangement. "It's impossible," she said. "She's in no condition to go to the hospital unless you take her in an ambulance and have her met at the emergency door with a wheelchair." She paused for a moment, then had a commonsense but fateful afterthought. "Oh, you don't have to do all that," she said. "There's a mobile lab that can come and check the blood at home. I'll call the doctor."

She made the call from her office; and, as she later told my daughter, "We did not exactly have a meeting of minds." She said she had told The Great Doctor that she would not be responsible for what happened if he insisted on having my wife go to the hospital; she reminded him that she had seen his patient twice—and he hadn't laid eyes on her yet. The discussion must have been acrimonious, for she told my daughter, calmly but positively, "I never want anything to do with *that* man again!"

She at least prodded The Great Doctor into action. He came tearing up to our house in his car about six-thirty that night. He talked to me for a few minutes by the front steps. He had had a chance by this time to study the report Dr. Ebert had mailed to him. "They found when they went in," he said, "that the valve was in much worse shape than we had thought. She could only have had a year or two to live without the operation, three at the most—and they wouldn't have been good years."

He asked me if Julia had always acted up as she was now doing, and I told him, no, she had originally been the most optimistic, cheery person in the world, but the successive shocks she had suffered while carrying this burden for seventeen years had reduced her to her present state. Evidently referring to the possibility of the heart-lung-machine gap, he said, "This is something that doesn't happen very often, and, unfortunately, it seems always to happen to those you least want it to."

Inside the house, he examined Julia carefully, but here again, as I later realized, the cult of the surgeon determined the nature of his examination and influenced his decision. His whole attention was concentrated on the plumbing. And that, he pronounced, was simply wonderful. Julia had a beautifully functioning valve; her chest and lungs were clear, her blood pressure good. The pallid appearance that had so alarmed Barbara's young friend made no impression on him.

(Later, Dr. Ebert, perhaps in attempted exculpation of a colleague, would suggest that The Great Doctor had had no basis for comparison. "He had not seen your wife before, had he?" he asked, meaning since the operation.

"No," I told him. But that, of course, is precisely the point: he should have seen her; he should not have been practicing medicine by telephone with a patient just come from open-heart surgery, and one who, in addition, was in obvious difficulties.)

After his examination of my wife, The Great Doctor lectured her. "Julia," he said, "you may think you are going to die, you many even want to die—but I'm not going to let you. I've got too much time and effort invested in this case, and I'm not going to let it happen."

He warned my wife that she would have to eat or he would put her in the hospital and force-feed her. "And you're not going to like that at all," he said, threateningly. Next, he said she had to exercise more. "There's no reason why you shouldn't be fully dressed by this time and sitting out under that tree in the yard," he told her, pointing outside. "You've got to get up off your ass and get moving."

He said he would go along this one time with having the mobile lab come to the house for the blood test, but he was obviously furious with the Public Health nurse who had dared to challenge him. "If that Public Health nurse gives me any more trouble," he said, "I'll boot her right off the case."

In two weeks, he said, he expected Julia to be well enough to follow his original schedule; he would accept no excuses then. In two weeks she was to go to the hospital for her blood test and then come over to his office for her examination. A two-week blood-testing schedule was obviously satisfactory to him.

Outside the house, he assured me that the results of the operation would exceed our most optimistic hopes. Since Julia had been able to do as much as she had with her valve in poor condition, the improvement now that her valve had been repaired so beautifully would be al-most phenomenal.

What I had no way of knowing at the time was that he was overlooking the most vital factor in the postopera-tive care of heart-surgery patients; I had no idea that he had no understanding of what he had just seen.

15

EARLY FRIDAY MORNING, THE GREAT DOCTOR'S
office telephoned. The Public Health Service's mobile lab
couldn't make the blood test that day; it would come on
Monday. There were, of course, a number of commer-
cial labs that would have sent someone to the house to
make the test, but The Great Doctor's secretary didn't
suggest this and I, knowing nothing about such arrangements, never thought of it.

"All right?" the secretary asked when she told me
about the postponement; and since it seemed all right
with her, I let it pass.

Friday was another night of restless horror, worse
than anything my wife had experienced since the night-
marish hallucinations early Wednesday morning. The
hallucinations were still bothering her, but they seemed
to have taken a milder form. She was now seeing moun-
tains and a blue lake; she remarked once that she saw a
whole line of cars and trucks in front of our house when,
in fact, the street was empty. These false images still unnerved her, made her wonder about her sanity; but they
did not seem to be the cause of her extreme restlessness
Friday night.

She complained that her body felt bruised and sore,
and that her skin felt tender all over. She tried the hos-

pital bed, she tried the couch; she even climbed the stairs to her second-story bedroom for the first time since she came home. But after five minutes, she said: "That's no good either. I'm going back downstairs even if I break my neck."

I helped her down. The sleeping pill seemed to have done nothing to quiet her; Valium didn't help. I knew that this could not go on.

Convinced now that my wife should be in the hospital, I telephoned The Great Doctor the first thing Saturday morning. I explained exactly what had happened the previous night. I told him that my wife seemed to me to be getting worse, that I didn't know how to cope with the situation, and that I felt certain she should be in the hospital.

The Great Doctor was in one of his most arrogant and snappish moods; but, to do him justice, he was a terribly overburdened man on this weekend. He had twenty-four patients in the hospital, plus the usual chaotic run of office problems; and when I urged him to admit Julia, he declared it was impossible.

"The only way I could get her in would be to put her in the psychiatric ward, and I don't want to do that," he said. "There isn't a bed to be had this weekend. I can't get anyone in unless it is a life-and-death emergency."

It reminded me of the day, less than a month before, that I had taken Julia into New York Hospital. No bed available. Nothing to be done. Would The Great Doctor have acted differently had there been room in the hospital? Would my wife's life have been saved?

Well, I asked, what was I to do?

"It's obviously too much for you," he said. "Can't your daughter help?"

I pointed out to him, a fact that he well knew, that

Barbara was a widow with three young children to care for; there wasn't much she could do.

"Well, what about the neighbors?" he asked. "Certainly you ought to be able to get some of the neighbors to help."

This was the point at which I gave up in disgust. The neighbors, for God's sake! I hung up and called Barbara. What she said, I will not repeat, but she went into action, got in touch with the nurses' registry, and made arrangements for nurses to come to the house on a 9:00 A.M.-to-5:00 P.M. shift for a week, beginning with the next day, Sunday.

When she called me back to tell me about this arrangement, she said: "Look, you've got to get away for a while. I'll get Linda to look after the boys, and I'll come down this afternoon and sit with mother. You go out in the boat or to the beach for a couple of hours."

This I did. When I came back, Julia seemed less distraught. She spent a quieter night Saturday, but I am not certain that she actually felt any better. She had the television on for the first time for a good part of the night, and I found her at times sitting on the couch supporting her head with her hands. I suspect she had decided that nothing was going to be done to help her and had simply resigned herself to the inevitable.

Sunday, another in that chain of Sundays, a registered nurse came to the house and stayed with Julia all day, trying to make her comfortable, bathing her, walking with her, cooking a noon meal for her. Julia seemed to feel a little better with the new attention; she ate fairly well at noontime. But by night she was turning away from food again.

About five-thirty, half an hour after the nurse left, Julia complained of a headache. This was something new, and I felt the first faint twinge of apprehension. Still, the headache did not seem to be too severe; and about seven o'clock I gave her Tylenol.

"Get well, dear," I told her as I gave her the pills, "and we'll go on a vacation up to New Hampshire in the fall."

Julia smiled at me faintly and began to doze in the large reclining chair we had moved into the dining room to make space for her hospital bed. I prepared my own supper and was eating it at the table, not far from where she slumbered, when she suddenly roused and called out, "I've got a splitting headache."

She put both hands to her head. I jumped up from the table and reached her in three strides; but in that instant her whole body seemed to go flaccid. I urged her to help herself by pushing down on the arm of the chair with one hand while I lifted her on the other side. She managed to do this, just barely, and I staggered with her to the hospital bed. Into this she collapsed, murmuring over and over: "Help me, help me. I'm going to die, I'm going to die."

In a panic, I telephoned Barbara. She summoned the first-aid service. While we were waiting, Julia's hands twitched and she murmured over and over, "Gotta get up, gotta get up." Then she lost consciousness. The first-aid men dashed in, administered oxygen, lifted her onto a stretcher, and sped off to the hospital.

There The Great Doctor's residents and nurses in the emergency ward did their best to save her; and there the great man himself finally put in an appearance. He came up to me, greatly worried, and asked if Julia had been getting any extra Coumadin.

"No," I told him, "I've been giving her all her medications, and she's been getting just the one five-milligram tablet a night the hospital prescribed."

"You're sure she didn't have some squirreled away somewhere?" he asked. "You're sure she couldn't have been sneaking some?"

If looks could have killed, the one my daughter gave him would have removed one great doctor from the world on the spot.

"You see the trouble is," he explained, "that her blood has been thinned out way too much. We try to keep the protime count stabilized around twenty-two, but hers is seventy-seven, and there's been seepage into the brain. I can't understand how it could have happened."

Later I checked the Coumadin the hospital had given me—a month's supply, thirty pills. Julia had had one a night for ten nights, and there were twenty pills left in the bottle.

For my wife, from the moment she had suffered that splitting headache, there was virtually no hope. The hospital residents, learning that she had had open-heart surgery only three weeks previously, expected her heart to collapse at any moment; but—a tribute to Dr. Ebert's surgical skill—it didn't. It kept pounding away until her condition was stabilized enough for her to be removed from the emergency room and placed in intensive care.

All the resources of the hospital were now thrown into the futile battle to undo the damage neglect had done. On the hospital's part, it was a magnificent effort. According to staff members, never in their recollection had so many nurses, residents, and specialists labored on one person. It was all too late, of course; and, as if some grim jester were making sport of us, the medical foul-ups continued.

When I phoned the hospital early Monday morning, the information desk told me my wife's condition was "fair." Reprieve. The miracle we had not dared to hope for must have happened during the night, we thought.

But when I double-checked later with The Great Doctor's office, I found there had been no miracle. My wife's condition was unchanged, critical; the doctor did not know how the hospital could possibly have reported "fair."

Then, on Monday afternoon, the doorbell rang. There stood a black woman technician in her white coat, with her tray of tubes and paraphernalia—the representative of Friday's immobile mobile laboratory, now reactivated and come to take my wife's blood count. It was too much. My nerves snapped, and I was brutal.

"Your patient," I told the young woman, "is now dying in intensive care in the hospital because you couldn't get here Friday to test her blood."

The poor girl looked as stunned as if I had hit her with a baseball bat. "What happened?" she asked, and I told her. She explained that, on Friday, there had been only one person on duty in the office. There was a rigid rule that the office must be kept open at all costs, and so no one could leave to make the blood test.

Early that evening, I went to the hospital to see Julia. I felt that I was saying good-bye to her. She lay there unconscious, a nurse beside her constantly siphoning off mucus that gathered in her throat. I took Julia's hand; it was cold to my touch, and she did not know, of course, that I was holding it. I looked down at her as she lay there, a faint reddish discoloration across her forehead above the eyebrows. The long surgical scar down her chest had healed beautifully and was already beginning to fade—and all for nothing. I knew without being told that she was dying.

The heart that Dr. Ebert had fixed so well kept pounding away for some thirty hours before it gave out around two-thirty A.M. on Tuesday, July 23. The operation that we had hoped would prolong Julia's life had cut it short.

Even then, the medical system could not right itself to get the plain fact of death straight. A lawyer neighbor of mine, worried about Julia, telephoned the hospital about six-thirty A.M. Though my wife had been dead for four hours, the cheery voice of the girl on the information desk told him that her condition was "fair."

In accordance with Julia's repeatedly expressed wishes, we held the funeral the next day; and on Thursday morning about ten-thirty I telephoned Dr. Ebert's office. I had already determined to investigate what had happened; to do something, if I could, to help prevent such needless tragedies from happening to others. It was, I had decided, the only possible compensation, the only thing that I could do for Julia now.

"Oh, how are you, Mr. Cook?" Dr. Ebert's secretary asked when I called.

"I'm all right," I told her. "But my wife isn't."

"Oh," the secretary asked, "what's the matter?"

"She's dead," I said.

There was an audible gasp on the phone, then the secretary asked, "What happened?" I explained.

Julia had now been dead for some fifty-six hours, but Dr. Ebert had been unaware until I called. Nobody had talked to anybody; the fact of death, it seemed, had not been all that important.

16

I MET HIM ON THE TRAIN THAT MONDAY MORNING, July 29, as I was going into New York to see Dr. Ebert. He was a stranger who was to become a friend, a man in his seventies, well and conservatively dressed, wearing a soft summer hat and a little bow tie. He was outgoing and friendly, sometimes garrulous, with lips that puckered with good humor as he related anecdotes from a busy life.

He had had a varied career, ranging from political dabbling to theatrical promotions. He had wound up as an executive in a large New York firm and now, semi-retired, he still kept a hand in various projects. On the train ride to the city, we exchanged experiences. I told him Julia's story; and here, at once, I discovered that my wife's tragic, unnecessary death touched a universal nerve.

After listening to me, he responded with a story of his own. It was one, like many others that were to come my way, that touched several basic themes: the way the cult of the surgeon so often blinds the medical profession to the life-threatening problems the surgeon himself creates; the need for skepticism and the employment of a layman's sound common sense to double-check on the oversights of the professionals; the lack of genuine care and compassion that so often leads workers in the system to blame the patient for not recovering instead of trying to analyze and understand the patient's problems; and, finally, the inestimable boon if a patient is fortunate enough to have a clear-eyed outsider with some basic knowledge who is able to deliver a kick in the pants to professional complacency.

My new friend was a bachelor who lived alone in a small midtown New York apartment. A few years previously, he had had a urinary blockage; he had gone into one of the great New York hospitals and had been operated on by a capable surgeon. His was the old story; the operation had been a success, but . . .

In his case, he knew himself he was not recovering as he should; indeed, he felt he was getting weaker day by day. He complained to his doctor, but the doctor brushed him off. His fears were ridiculous, he was told; he had come through the operation in great style. All he had to do now was go home, rest, and recuperate.

And so he had returned to his bachelor's quarters where there was no one to take care of him. There, as the days passed, he continued to feel weaker and weaker.

"Finally," he said, "this one morning, I got up and I could hardly stand. I thought I was going to pass out on the floor. Somehow—I'll never know quite how I managed to do it—I succeeded in getting myself dressed, and I staggered down to the street and hailed a cab. 'Take me to the hospital,' I told the cabbie."

His doctor was amazed to find him back in a hospital bed. "What is the matter with you?" he asked.

"Well, doctor," my friend replied, "I kept telling you I was feeling worse, and this morning I almost passed out on the floor."

The hospital began to give him tests. He noticed

that his feces had a peculiar, tarlike color, and he pointed this out to a nurse, who shrugged the symptom off as being of no consequence. The tests he was given failed to disclose anything wrong with him, but his debilitating weakness continued.

It was at this point that a friend came to his rescue. The friend had had some serious health problems, had read widely in medical literature, and so had some idea of what should be done. "My friend asked me if I had had a certain test—I forget the name of it now—but, anyway, I hadn't had it," the former patient said.

The next time he saw his doctor, he asked about this particular test. "Oh, you don't need that," he was told.

"Well, doctor, I'm told I should have it, and I'm going to get out of this hospital today."

"You can't do that. I won't release you."

"Doctor, you didn't understand me. I just fired you, and I'm signing myself out."

He did. His friend got him a new internist. He was placed in another hospital, and there the new expert quickly determined what was wrong with him.

"The test showed," he said, "that as a result of the trauma of the surgery I had developed what is known as a 'stress' ulcer. It is something that doesn't happen often, but it did in my case. Why it did, I don't know, because I had never had even a hint of such a problem before. But there it was. I was bleeding away internally, and I could have died if it hadn't been for the friend who suspected what was happening and got me a new doctor."

He was operated on a second time for the ulcer, recovered, and now seems in the best of health—thanks to the independent, lay advice that corrected the oversights of the medical system in time to prevent another tragedy.

The magazine article I was soon to write after my

interview with Dr. Ebert would lance a common boil, and a spate of similar experiences would pour forth, varying only in detail. One that dovetails in many respects with the near-miss suffered by my new friend was told to me in a detailed, eight-page account written by Mrs. Jean Marks, of 70 East Ninety-sixth Street, New York.

Her father and mother, living on a farm near Charlottesville, Virginia, were involved in an automobile accident on a Friday in early May, 1969. Her father was unhurt, but her mother, then seventy-four, sitting in the front seat beside him, was thrown violently forward. Mrs. Marks wrote that "her glasses were broken, she had facial and arm bruises and three broken ribs."

She was taken to the University of Virginia Hospital, where apparently "all the right things were done in admitting her." X rays were taken; they seemed to show that the only serious injury was the broken ribs, and a chest expert was put in charge of her case. "A friend here who had graduated from UVA's medical school confirmed Dr. X's reputation; he could get in and out of a chest faster than any surgeon on the East Coast."

Mrs. Marks bundled up her two small children and went to Charlottesville to take care of her father. They made daily twenty-mile trips to the hospital to see her mother, who at first seemed "quite cheerful." She was able to walk, was eating well "and congratulating herself on not being more seriously hurt."

During the second week in the hospital, however, Mrs. Marks's mother "began to complain of headaches." Whatever treatment she was given did not seem to help. "During the next week," Mrs. Marks wrote, "she began to cry when I entered the room, saying that she had bubbles in her head and that she was afraid she was losing her mind." No doctor was on the floor at these times, but

Mrs. Marks discussed her mother's worsening condition with the nurses.

Later, Mrs. Marks's sister, Sarah, spoke to one of the residents. "He knew, he said, of my mother's complaints, and we were not to worry. She was doing fine; the ribs were healing, and she would be released shortly. She *was* depressed, he said, but that was not uncommon in a woman of her age."

Despite such comforting reassurances, Mrs. Marks's mother continued to fail. A neighbor who visited her in the hospital during the dinner hour one day found her unable to get food to her mouth and started to feed her. Then "a nurse entered the room ordering our neighbor to stop, saying: 'She's just feeling sorry for herself; she has to learn to do that herself.'"

Mrs. Marks found, just as I had, that the tension and worry of the time made one day merge into another, so that it became difficult to remember later just when certain things had happened, though the highlights remained indelible in memory. She wrote:

> Was this when an intern accused her of being on Medicare and not wanting to go home? Was this when antidepressant pills were prescribed? For this woman? The one who came from a genteel urban life to the country, who learned to cook on a wood stove—in August for field hands, not country chic—the one who drew water from a well to heat in the copper boiler on the wood stove for every Monday morning's wash for twenty years; the one who canned and preserved, who learned how to make soap and sew and clean the lampshades and chamber pots, nurse and raise five children and care for a father-in-law. That one who had learned about raising chickens to help send her children to

college. . . . Antidepressant pills for broken ribs? Old age? An accident? For that generation of woman? Malingering?

Mrs. Marks's mother continued to get worse. "She lay in bed most of the time, she couldn't get to the bathroom by herself; it now took two people to carry her. When she talked, it was with great effort. She cried. She couldn't use her right hand at all. I was becoming frightened."

A staff doctor told her that her mother was being taken off medication and would start physical therapy the following week. "It takes time for older people," he said. When Mrs. Marks repeated this to a neighbor, Pearl Chapman, the latter shook her head and said, "No, your mother is dying; she has a slow leak in her head."

Jolted by this frank opinion, Mrs. Marks sent out an alarm to all members of the family. Edith, another of her sisters who, she writes, is "often an angry woman," stormed into the hospital and took charge. "She began at the nurses' station, and she never took a backward step." The nurses accused the family of becoming hysterical. "You're Goddamned right I'm hysterical," Edith boomed in tones that could have been heard clear up to Monticello. "My mother is dying. She was in better shape four weeks ago. Why didn't you leave her by the side of the road? No, I'll wait. I don't want to talk to him or him or you [pointing]; I want to see Dr. X."

By the time Dr. X made himself available, the whole family clan had gathered, down even to nephews and nieces. Dr. X said he would see just two members of the delegation. "If he spoke, we didn't hear him," Mrs. Marks wrote. The only voice that came through the office wall was that of her sister, "and she was not being nice." She was shouting, "By God, I'll sue."

The next day, "our mother went into a coma." Panic now in the hospital. Doctors asked and were given permission to operate. "They shaved her head, drilled holes in her skull to release the blood trapped inside." The neighborhood farm woman had been right, and Mrs. Marks is convinced that, except for her jolting intervention, her mother would probably have died.

With the pressure on the brain relieved, Mrs. Marks's mother, a determined and courageous woman, fought her way through the physical therapy regime and recovered. "She will be eighty this April," Mrs. Marks wrote in February, 1975, six years after the operation. "She cares for herself, my father and their home by herself. They have been good years, she says, six very good years."

The ordeal led Mrs. Marks to form a set of conclusions about the operation of the medical system as she had observed it. Some of her observations duplicate my own, and many are reflected again and again in letters I have received and the accounts of persons I have interviewed. They apply, it seems, not to just one great hospital or one great doctor, but to many.

Mrs. Marks, just as we did, for a long time accepted what the medical experts told her. "I didn't listen to—I didn't *hear* my mother," she wrote. She continued:

> The Great Doctor neither looked at nor listened to his patient after his original diagnosis was made; the nursing staff's first reaction to things not going well was punitive; no one talked—communicated—with anyone else, doctor to patient, doctor to patient's family, doctor on the case to the family doctor; the only [people whose] vision . . . stayed clear were the "unedu-

cated," the "unsophisticated": my old neighbor and hospital aides looked and saw; the aides often seemed to me to be the only people at the hospital who were *caring* for my mother. And from what I saw of that rigid power hierarchy, no one speaks to an aide.

17

IT WAS A GUILT-BURDENED MAN WHO MADE THAT dreary walk in summer heat from the IRT subway through the squalid East Side streets, where one caught an occasional whiff of someone smoking pot, along the blocks separating the avenues down to New York Hospital, up the wide circular driveway to the entrance door, into the high-vaulted hall and down the long corridor. I had made that trip many times in this disastrous summer; I had made it in dread, in relief, in buoyant optimism, convinced that an Elysian future would be ours. Now I made it in grim despair, hating myself.

We all felt guilt, everyone who had been close to Julia, everyone who had knowledge of the case. I had reason to feel it, but others did not. The others had done their best, and could not have been expected to do more; but they still felt out of compassion and love that they should have done more, that they, too, should share the blame.

It was useless for Barbara to say, however basically right she may have been: "Dad, you *must* stop blaming yourself. It wasn't your fault. We're not professional people; we're not supposed to know. It was *their* fault—and no one else's." She could tell me this, and yet blame herself, too. As she would say on another occasion, "Linda *told* me. Why didn't I scream and stamp my feet and *demand* that something be done?" She hadn't, of course, because almost at the same time Linda told her, The Great Doctor examined Julia and pronounced her "fine." And Linda, that most perceptive girl, who *had* told Barbara, who *had* done all anyone could ever have expected of her, would still feel that she should have done more. "I *knew* what was happening," she said months later. "I even called it to the day. Why didn't I scream and yell and *do* something?"

Even Margaret Edelson, that invaluable friend—the most sympathetic and understanding person, marvelous in her courage and common sense—felt an unnecessary twinge. "I feel a sense of guilt, too," she told me sometime after Julia's death. "Julia called me, and I know now that she was asking for help. And all I did was what everyone else did. I tried to soothe her and pat her on the head verbally and assure her everything was going to be all right. But all the doctors had said she was 'fine,' and I thought they knew what they were talking about."

Neither she nor any of the others, I am convinced, had any real reason for self-reproach. With me, it was different. I have been a journalist all my life; I know how to research, how to investigate difficult situations. Why hadn't *I* in all those years taken the trouble really to study the literature on the multiple problems posed by open-heart surgery? Why had I put such blind faith in the experts who were supposed to know? I had even written a book, *The Plot Against the Patient*, exposing many of the flaws in the disorganized medical and hospital system. And then I had acted the credulous fool, naïvely assuming that, if you really got *the best*, the best wouldn't let you down.

Ten years before, I had known something about Coumadin, not what I believe now every person taking it should know, but enough to make me apprehensive; and so in the hospital, on that terrible Sunday night, when I learned that Coumadin had been the secret villain, I felt as if a mule had kicked the guts right out of me. *If* I had remembered what I once had known, my wife's life in all probability could have been saved despite the medical profession; but I, who had loved her and might have saved her, had forgotten everything.

The instant I was told that Coumadin had thinned Julia's blood to a fatal degree, my mind flashed back to the briefing Dr. Economos had given us when she left George Washington University Hospital for that brief Coumadin-taking period in 1964. I had had no idea even then that Coumadin could be lethal, but Dr. Economos had been emphatic in warning us that Julia's blood must be checked regularly every seven days. From what he said, I had gotten the uneasy impression that this might be a very tricky drug, and I had been concerned enough to write a friend, then an assistant administrator in one of the smaller New York hospitals, inquiring whether Coumadin was safe. He had replied that it was a drug used all the time for a variety of ailments and that, if a careful check was kept, we should have no problem. Nor did we. I suppose that, because everything had gone so smoothly then, I had put the whole experience out of my mind in the intervening ten years; and that ever-so-casual briefing in New York Hospital had not been enough to trigger recollection. I knew all the excuses that could be made for me—and that my family and friends tried to make— but I could not forgive myself.

It was in this mood that I saw Dr. Ebert. He was his usual soft-voiced, compassionate self. "Mr. Cook," he said at the outset, "I'm sorry about what happened to your wife. I had not expected that."

He said that, after his office received my call, he had checked with The Great Doctor, who confirmed that runaway Coumadin had caused my wife's death. Dr. Ebert had been much surprised, he said, because when Julia had been put on Coumadin in the hospital immediately after the operation, her blood had stabilized almost at once, and it had remained stable during daily blood checks for twelve consecutive days. "There was no sign of a problem," he said.

What, then, had happened? He could hazard only a theory. Sometimes, he said, when a patient has suffered a heart impairment for so long, the lack of oxygen in the system causes hidden liver damage. Perhaps my wife's liver (the liver is the only organ that forms platelets, small disks that aid in blood clotting) had begun to malfunction, failing to produce enough platelets to keep the Coumadin in balance. Medical literature, however, agrees that the mitral-valve operation, by restoring the oxygen supply, "usually" corrects such liver problems; and, as Dr. Ebert assured me, there had been no indication of a liver inadequacy in Julia's case during her stay in the hospital. He acknowledged that, if a protime blood test had been taken in time, her life could have been saved.

"But she had had her blood tested after she went home, hadn't she?" he asked.

"No," I told him.

"Oh," he said.

I indicated to him that I thought the hospital had been remiss in its casual Coumadin briefing. Instead of referring to some vague and meaningless "periodic" blood count, why couldn't the printed instructions have been specific? It seemed to me that they should have emphasized the matter: "It is *important* that your blood be checked every seven days during the early recuperative period after you return home."

Well, Dr. Ebert replied, not all doctors check the blood that frequently, (there is, as I was to find out, absolutely no excuse for them if they don't), and the hospital preferred to leave such things to the judgment of "the family doctor." Professional courtesy seemed to be the paramount consideration. But, as I told him, all I had needed was a simple, pointed reminder; if I had gotten it, "I damn well would have had my wife's blood checked on time, doctor or no doctor."

Dr. Ebert wondered whether, even if this had been done, "the end result would have been much different." He explained that he had been disturbed by my wife's obvious depression when he first examined her. He would much rather operate any day, he said, on a patient whose heart might be much worse than hers but whose psychological attitude was better. Cases like Julia's, he said, are the ones that give him the greatest anxiety because, if a patient's mind is fixed on death, he or she is "going to accomplish it one way or another."

He explained that this is a syndrome he encounters most frequently in persons between fifty-five and sixty-five who have borne the burden of heart trouble for a long time. Younger persons, full of optimism about the future, wanting life, present no such psychological problems. Nor, peculiarly enough, do older patients in their seventies. "I do not know why this is," Dr. Ebert said, "but perhaps it's that they've had to be tough to have lived so long and they get the feeling they're tough enough to stand anything."

As an example of the destruction mental attitudes can cause, he cited what he called "Class 4 cases." These are persons who have had open-heart surgery because their doctors and their families have convinced them that they must; physically, they have been restored to health, but they remain helpless invalids confined to wheelchairs. "We can bring them in here," Dr. Ebert said, "and give them catheterizations and the most sophisticated tests; and we find their valves are functioning perfectly, their hearts are fine, their chests and lungs are clear. But there they sit, convinced they're helpless, and there's nothing you can do to convince them they aren't."

Many patients, he said, go into the operation prepared to die; then they wake up in intensive care, find they have survived, and "are not prepared for life and its problems." In my wife's case, he seemed to feel that her state of mind would have doomed her in the long run. She had told him what she had told me: "I know I'm not going to make it. I know I'm going to die." He said that he had tried to talk her out of this attitude. "She seemed to be doing well," he said. "She never complained very much of pain, much less than most patients, and she seemed glad everything went well. But still she didn't seem to believe us when we told her she was going to get better. I sat down and tried to convince her that in a few months—three perhaps, or six at the most—she would feel better than she had felt in years. But I felt I wasn't making any impression."

I suggested, acknowledging that this was hindsight, that it might have been better to send my wife back to our local hospital instead of sending her home. "I don't like to do that usually," Dr. Ebert said. "I find it's not good for patients psychologically to be sent from one hospital to another. They begin to wonder whether something is seriously wrong with them. I've found it's much better usually to send them back to their own homes, where they can have their family, friends, and home things around them. If they are going to snap out of it, they usually will there, and that's what I expected would happen in your wife's case." It was, he added, "very uncommon for us to get a call that a patient has done worse at home."

Perhaps so, but I am convinced that there were many things Dr. Ebert, great surgeon that he is, simply did not comprehend. He was right in his assessment of my wife's profound depression when he first met her, but he was wrong in thinking she was death-motivated. He had no knowledge of the change he himself had wrought in her. He did not see the buoyant optimism with which she faced the operation as a result of her confidence in him; he could not know that she had asked the director of her heart association whether she might possibly get back to work in a month because she did not want someone else doing her job.

I am convinced that Julia went into the operation very much wanting to live. There is a vast difference between being death-motivated and being psychically possessed by a premonition that death is going to come somehow. Many heart patients, I was to learn, experience such dire presentiments in the postoperative period, but in most cases these recede as the patient gets stronger. In my wife's case, this did not happen, largely because of the persistence of those hallucinations that so disturbed her mind. I could never be certain how aware Dr. Ebert was of this factor, how complete were the communications between the floor personnel and the cardiologists; but I got the impression that there was a tendency to dismiss such manifestations—like my wife's morning "crying spells"—as relatively inconsequential when the operation itself had been so successful and the physical signs seemed so good. Though the deep psychological trauma of such surgery is recognized by doctors, inadequate attention seems to have been paid to the problem. Soothing reassurance, as we found out ourselves, simply was not enough.

At the outset of my interview with Dr. Ebert, I showed him a five-page, single-spaced letter that I had written to a friend in Florida outlining in considerable detail what had happened. He reacted strongly to only one item in it: that "bubbles in my head" phrase. We in the family had laughed at this at the time, but I learned soon after Julia's death that she had not been fanciful in this description. Experienced residents and nurses who have handled heart-surgery patients assured me that Julia had given a very precise description of what she was feeling. The "bubbles in my head" expression is one that professionals have heard innumerable times. It indicates either brain damage from a heart-lung-machine gap or pressures on the brain from some other cause; definitely, it is no laughing matter.

I got the distinct impression that Dr. Ebert first became aware of Julia using this phrase when he read my letter; it was the one thing that seemed to surprise him, the one thing to which he reacted instantly.

"With the type of filters we're using now," he said, "I don't see how any air bubbles could have gotten into her blood."

He also doubted that the explanation was a heart-lung-machine gap. If this had been the cause of the trouble, he reasoned, those horror images that had so shaken Julia that early Wednesday morning should have developed much earlier, while she was in the hospital. In addition, he said, brain damage in such instances almost always causes a blurring of vision; and he related how he had found Julia sitting up in bed one morning, reading a newspaper. (This came as a shock to me because, with the family, she had pretended to be unable to read her get-well cards.) "Read me a couple of sentences," Dr. Ebert said he had asked. He added: "And she did. She read me two or three sentences, not very much, but she read them clearly and obviously was having no trouble with her eyesight."

Such was the interview. As I left, Dr. Ebert said to me: "Mr. Cook, you are understandably bitter. But don't let it destroy you, too. You have to go on, you know."

Yes, I know.

18

THE DIRECTORS OF TWO COUNTY HEART ASSOCIATIONS were talking on the telephone, both appalled by what they hadn't known. One had just read the November 18, 1974, issue of *New York* magazine, which had devoted its entire cover to a display of the article I had written about Julia's case. As she read, this heart-association director had become horrified; what shocked her most was that, closely involved in heart work though she was, she had no idea of the problems connected with heart operations.

She had never heard of such hallucinations, nor had the other director, despite years of heart-association work. No doctor had ever mentioned anything about it to either of them.

The first director was worried. Wasn't this a reflection on the heart association itself? The second director said she didn't think so; the reflection, as she saw it, was on the medical profession for being so secretive. The two directors continued to discuss the situation at some length, and one of them, in telling me about it later, said, "What gets me is that here we are so deeply involved in heart work, and we find ourselves sitting out on the periphery, knowing virtually nothing."

It was a highly revealing incident, shedding its own

light on one of the fundamental flaws in the chaotic medical system—the failure to communicate, the stubborn refusal to tell patients and others what they have a right to know, what they *have* to know.

American doctors, like pagan medicine men, take the attitude that only they have the right to The Knowledge. The patient is supposed to know nothing, to leave everything to them—never to question, just to do what he is told. This is a prescription for disaster. With a medical profession too overburdened or too indifferent to make house calls and keep a close check on patients, it is more vital than ever that the patients and their families become knowledgeable partners in the process of care. They cannot deal with situations that confront them if they do not know what they are confronted with; and, in these circumstances, keeping vital information from them only insures that there will continue to be thousands of needless deaths.

In our case, Julia's hallucinations drove her into an emotional frenzy that may well have played its part in the overreaction to Coumadin. Neither she nor any of the rest of us in the family were prepared for this; had we been, had the great hospital or The Great Doctor paid any real attention to the problem, the trauma might well have been less severe.

There can be no excuse, it seems to me, for two dedicated heart-association directors being kept in ignorance of one of the most common and threatening postoperative problems in open-heart surgery. *Most* heart patients suffer the shock of unnerving hallucinations. Many have told me about seeing purple monsters climbing the walls, or about becoming positively paranoid, convinced doctors and nurses were plotting to kill them. These aberrations usually disappear in a few days, often by the time the patient is ready to leave intensive care, and medical literature indicates that they should be "transitory." This certainly was not so in my wife's case, and that in itself, it would seem, should have been a warning signal.

In the family, we did not know what we were dealing with in the beginning; and even after we were given some belated, partial knowledge, we had little grasp of the situation, little understanding of its potential danger. Yet the whole subject has been clearly dealt with in medical literature, as I discovered in a few hours' research in the New York Academy of Medicine after my wife died.

The American College of Surgeons in 1971 published a volume entitled *Manual of Preoperative and Postoperative Care*. Dr. W. Gerald Austin, professor of surgery at Harvard Medical School and chief of surgery at Massachusetts General Hospital, wrote in an article entitled "Cardiac Surgery":

> Psychological problems are *very common* following cardiac surgery. The emotional stress of a life-and-death situation, the rigors of the postoperative period in an intensive care unit, and perhaps a number of other unrecognized factors result in various psychological conditions. Depression, visual and auditory hallucinations, agitation, disorientation and paranoid delusion are *common problems*. [Italics added.]

Even patients who have given "no previous evidence of psychological difficulties" develop such problems, Dr. Austin wrote, and he added that this psychological turmoil is most severe among older patients (like my wife) who have borne the depressing burden of illness for a considerable time.

Other evidence indicates that the heart-lung machine, even when it functions without flaw, often causes the kind of brain damage that leads to such psychological aberrations. *Science Digest* reported in January, 1975:

> It is known that as blood passes through the pump, there is some destruction of red blood cells. One study using an ultrasonic detector also has demonstrated that all commercially available oxygenerators generate blood clots. Microscopic examinations of the brains of patients at autopsy have shown multiple small lesions distributed through the gray and white matter.

Bubbles in the head, indeed!

Despite the recognition of the potential seriousness of such postoperative psychological traumas, the medical profession as a whole does practically nothing to prepare the patient or the patient's family for the problems with which, in all probability, they are going to have to cope. Perhaps the most significant study in this area was made in 1972 by Dr. Chase Patterson Kimball, a researcher for Yale University Medical School. In a six-year study of 200 open-heart surgery cases, Dr. Kimball found that *at least 70 percent* of the patients had experienced psychological aftereffects.

These included temporary loss of memory and intellectual function, delusions, and even life-threatening depressions. Many patients became withdrawn, depressed, and convinced that neither the operation nor the care they were getting would be of the slightest benefit. One fifty-year-old man was unable to comprehend a single sentence; another, fifty-seven, went berserk, shouting incoherently and trying to rise and tear the intravenous tube from his arm.

Dr. Kimball concluded that oxygen deprivation during surgery appeared to explain only a handful of such reactions. Most mental disturbances, he thought, were emotional in origin, and he argued with seemingly irrefutable logic that such psychological upheavals, which sometimes retard and even prevent recovery, could be reduced and brought under better control if more care were taken *before* surgery. He advocated thorough briefing of patients and their families about what sometimes happens when a patient comes out of anesthesia. This advance warning, something that is rarely provided, could reduce the emotional anguish, he thought, and enable the patient to cope better with experiences that otherwise would be unnerving and horrifying. In my wife's case, psychological preparation might have relieved her of the conviction that she was going insane; certainly, reassurance *after* the event did no good.

One who was fortunate enough to get this kind of briefing before surgery is the husband of a plump, good-natured woman who used to sing with Julia in the church choir. We had never been close friends of the couple; and, unfortunately, we had not talked with them before Julia went in for surgery. The husband—let's call him Walter; her, Ruth—is a retired army sergeant who had had two serious heart attacks and needed bypass surgery. This is a procedure in which a vein is taken from the leg and used to re-route the blood around the damaged, deadened sections of the heart. The operation has come into its own only in the last few years and is much more complicated than the mitral-valve replacement my wife had. After being treated for his heart attacks in a local base hospital, Walter was sent to Walter Reed Army Medical Center in Washington, D.C., in early May, 1973.

He was in the hospital five days before the operation was performed, a period that was spent in the most meticulous preparation. There was none of the rush-rush procedure so common in large metropolitan hospitals. The chief cardiac nurse, a cardiologist on the operating team, and finally the chief surgeon himself all took detailed case histories of the patient, then met and compared notes to make certain nothing had been missed. Walter was shown the operating room and the intensive care unit; he was allowed to walk around the hospital and talk to other patients who had come through heart surgery and were recuperating. This was an encouraging procedure.

Ruth feels that the only reason her husband is alive today is that such care was taken both before and after the operation; she is convinced that he wouldn't have survived anywhere else. Even so, even in this hospital where the emphasis was on taking time and doing everything right, there was a peculiar blind spot regarding postoperative trauma.

Fortunately, Ruth had worked for several years in a state hospital and had come to know the doctors well. One of them had undergone open-heart surgery twice and was facing it a third time. This grim ordeal was fairly common with the early valves, for in many instances they would give out after only five years, and then the patient, to survive, had to go through the entire grueling procedure again.

Knowing Ruth, the doctor who had survived two operations gave her his literature on open-heart surgery and briefed her on the psychological difficulties her husband might experience after he came out of anesthesia. So forewarned, Walter and Ruth went into the final conference with the surgeon who was to do the operation.

The doctor demonstrated, using a plastic heart, just what they were going to do, a briefing very similar to the one my wife was given in New York Hospital. Ruth waited to see what else he would say, but the surgeon obviously intended to end the briefing with this description of the physical procedure. Nothing was said about postoperative trauma—and so Ruth brought up the point.

"The surgeon looked at me," she said afterward, "as much as to say, 'What is this I've got on my hands?' But then he recognized that I wasn't a drooling idiot, that I wasn't going to become hysterical, and that I already knew something. And so he told us. But the point is that he wasn't going to, he wouldn't have, if I hadn't brought it up."

Walter went into the operation in a very calm frame of mind. He was fatalistic. "He took the attitude," Ruth says, "that, if he didn't have the operation, he probably would have only two or three months more to live anyway, so what difference did it make? If the operation succeeded, fine; if it didn't, he hadn't lost all that much."

Ruth says that the nurses told her afterward that her husband was the best patient they had ever had. And yet even this calm, controlled, courageous man became positively paranoid after surgery. "I was scared to death of the nurses," he told me. "I felt that people were laughing at me."

Ruth recalls that she was sitting at his bedside one day when a group of residents and interns came to examine him. Afterward, they drew off to a corner of the room, consulting among themselves in low voices.

"Look at that!" Walter exclaimed. "Look at that! They're plotting to kill me."

"Oh, Walt, you know that's ridiculous," Ruth told him. "Remember what we told you about this before the operation?"

He thought for a moment. "Yes," he said, "that's right." And that was the end of it.

There was, however, still something this well-briefed, well-informed couple hadn't been told. Walter recovered rapidly; he was released from the hospital seventeen days after the operation and came home. But then, in the next year and a half, up to the time I talked to him, he found that he was no longer able to function sexually.

"There's a group of us," Ruth says, "who call ourselves 'cardiac virgins.' The doctors seem to feel that the cause is largely psychological. Apparently many men, having gone through this terribly painful surgery, worry subconsciously about their hearts and are afraid the strain of sex will be too much for them. So they become impotent."

When Ruth realized that she had an incomplete husband, she was shocked and consulted with a friend whose husband had had open-heart surgery a year or so previously. She found that she was by no means alone.

The friend told her, she says, "Well, Ruth, you have just two choices: amputate or deviate."

Recalling this, Ruth says, "I cracked up. I laughed until I cried, with the tears running down my cheeks. Then I decided I didn't like either of those choices, and I'd stay. After all, if a marriage means anything, there's a lot more to it than sex."

Calmly as she takes the situation now, she is furious about the medical profession's fetish of secrecy; about the obstinate refusal to prepare patients and their families psychologically for the postoperative difficulties they may have to face.

"The thing is that no effort is made to prepare the wives for this possibility," Ruth says angrily. "It bursts on them out of the blue; they are not prepared for it, and it's very, very difficult for them to deal with. I feel strongly about this—that something should be done about it.

"It's just a damn shame that Julia had to die to bring some of this out into the open, but perhaps, this way, some good will come of it."

19

One of many letters came from a woman in Rye, New York. Having just read my magazine article about Julia's death, she wrote: "It brought up old memories of an episode that my husband had when he was put on Coumadin, was not properly followed [up] and almost died from internal hemorrhaging. . . . It is inconceivable to me that doctors treating such life-threatening situations should be so ignorant. I am sorry to say that I feel these deaths occur too often. . . ."

Another woman wrote from Sea Cliff, New York, that her husband had had a stroke, had been admitted to a hospital, treated, and discharged. She added: "He was released with a 'blood-thinning' medicine and aspirin and *no* instructions to see anyone again. Just a bottle of pills. My instincts told me that you just can't keep taking these, and after your article I've insisted he see his doctor again . . . hopefully we will keep tabs on his blood. Thank you for that."

A professional woman in Liberty, New York, described her experience with phlebitis, the clot-in-vein illness that almost killed ex-President Nixon. As is customary in such cases, she was placed on blood-thinning Coumadin. "I was told to have a blood test in a rather casual way," she wrote. Then she began to notice "little red marks on my feet. That was the thin blood seeping through. Also my monthly period was so bad I had to have shots for that, too, so it seems they try to cure one thing and destroy you with the same cure. . . ."

A widow in Flushing, New York, described the operation performed on her husband in December, 1973. He had been taken into a hospital for treatment of a blood clot. There it was discovered that he had an aneurysm (a weakening and bulging of the wall) of the aorta. Open-heart surgery was performed on the aorta; her husband survived it, recovered, and was sent home "without proper follow-up care. Our competent doctors never prescribed further anticoagulant pills," though blood-thinning medication is essential in such heart operations to keep blood clots from forming. In this instance, the patient was scheduled to have a blood test in early July, but the long Fourth of July holiday disrupted the schedule and the test was delayed. The result: he suffered a severe stroke, was hospitalized, had another stroke—and in August, 1974, he died.

A retired businessman from Rumson, New Jersey, sat in my study for two hours, describing the multiple ordeals of his sixty-five-year-old wife. It was a horror tale, ranging from a faulty first operation to inadequate briefing on postoperative treatment with, again, only passing attention paid to the blood factor. At the outset of our discussion, my guest, an obviously intelligent and capable person, capsuled his impressions in these words: "It's the system that is at fault. The doctors have come to be considered sacred cows, and the patient and the patient's family are just supposed to follow along, ask no questions, leave everything to them." It was a summation that struck a responsive chord in me; for, of course, we had done just that—and Julia had died.

My visitor was a short, solidly built man, deliberate

in his speech. He was torturing himself, as I had tortured myself, with all those second-guessing "ifs": if he had done *this* differently, if he had not done *that*, might she have lived?

His wife, he explained, had had several serious health problems from which she had recovered; but, first in February, then in May, 1973, she suffered two severe heart attacks. Her cardiologists decided she must have open-heart surgery and sent her to one of the great Pennsylvania university hospitals—ironically, the very hospital to which some second-guessers had told me I might have done better to take my wife.

The first operation seemed initially to justify the high estimates that are heard of this particular institution. The surgeons had to work on a severely damaged heart in a most complicated procedure. They had to install two bypasses, ream out a third artery, and replace the mitral valve. "She came through it all with flying colors," the husband said.

The operation was performed on December 4, 1973; his wife came home on December 21. She was weak, but she seemed to feel better than she had in a long time. It was a glorious Christmas. Then, shortly after the first of the year, the wife began to fail alarmingly.

She was taken to a local hospital, where she stayed for three weeks before doctors decided that she was having some mysterious leakage around the new mitral valve. They recommended she return to the hospital where the surgery had been done.

The new examination in the university hospital resulted in a horrifying discovery: the mitral valve had been anchored in bad tissue and was now pulling loose. "I never did find out why they sutured the valve into bad tissue," the husband said. "I never got any explanation of what went wrong in that first operation."

It was obvious that only one thing could be done now: a second open-heart operation to correct the error of the first. There was, however, a complication: the patient had picked up an infection and was running a 104° fever. Antibiotics brought the fever down, but her temperature was still not back to normal when the surgeons decided the valve was in such critical condition that they could delay no longer. And so, in early February, 1974, less than two months after she had been released from the hospital the first time, the wife was rushed back into the operating room.

By some miracle, she survived it; but when she was brought into intensive care, her worried husband became aware that there was consternation among the operating team. A sponge was missing.

The chief surgeon, very worried, explained that the wife had gone into cardiac arrest after the operation; they had had to massage her heart vigorously to get it functioning again; and in the tension of the moment, hurrying to close her up and get her into intensive care, they had not discovered that, while they had used thirteen sponges during the operation, they could now account for only twelve. "I hope it isn't in her," the surgeon said. It was: and so it was back in the operating room to snip a few stitches and get the sponge out.

The wife survived all this, just barely. She was now in distressing condition. She was hagridden by hallucinations and fantasies. She began to talk about a couple they hadn't seen in years as if she were inviting them over for dinner. She saw horrible purple monsters. "Everything seemed to be colored purple," her husband says. "They tell you nothing about things like this in advance, and you're not prepared for it." He questioned one of the doctors, who, he says, told him: "Don't worry. This is nothing unusual. Why, I saw one fellow who had a complete change of personality after the operation, but that was a year ago and he's all right now. Don't worry about it."

Just as Julia had, his wife rejected food; just as I had, he urged her to eat, saying, "You can't get your strength back without eating something." But she was nauseous and would not. Her weight fell from 140 to 104 pounds; she was so weak she could not walk. Yet, little improved, she was discharged from the hospital on March 22, 1974. "She has hospitalitis," a doctor told her husband. "She's not doing well at all. I think you better take her home and see if you can do something for her there."

At home there was, indeed, a very slow improvement; and in mid-May she and her husband went to a vacation home they owned in the Poconos. She was on a three-day Coumadin schedule: 2.5 milligrams the first two days, 5 milligrams the third, then a repetition of the sequence. There had been insufficient warning about Coumadin; they had been unaware of the need for frequent protime blood tests. "When I took her to a doctor in Tafton, Pennsylvania, for a checkup," the husband said, "he asked me what her doctors wanted her protime count stabilized at, and I asked him, 'What is a protime count?' I had never heard of it."

Their only warning had come from their local cardiologist before they left for the Poconos. The cardiologist had explained that, since the wife had been on Coumadin so long, there was a possibility of the blood's thinning too much, and one of the first signs of this might be discoloration of the stool. This, indeed, happened in early fall, just at a time when everything seemed to be going particularly well for them, and the husband took his wife to a nearby hospital, where she was placed in intensive care.

Her blood seemed to be acting up badly in two disparate ways. On the one hand, it had thinned out too much; on the other, there was evidence of clots. Hospital experts decided that the clots might have been caused by a bursting polyp; they recommended that the wife go back to the university hospital in which she had had her operations for a checkup. The doctor in charge of her case said, however, that there was no need to hurry. Since it would probably take him a week to get his report to the other hospital, if she went back in two weeks there would be time enough. It was a fatal miscalculation.

The couple returned to their home in the Poconos, and at 3:45 the next morning the husband woke to find his wife dead in bed, apparently the victim of a blood clot that had broken loose and hit the heart.

Such tragic experiences clearly demonstrate the critical importance of the blood factor in open-heart surgery, yet there seems to be a total misconception on the part of patients and much of the medical profession about where the greatest danger lies. The most critical life-and-death crisis comes, as I am convinced after listening to many such harrowing tales, not during surgery in the operating room but after the surgery has been performed and the patient has left the hospital. The operating technique itself has been perfected to the point where, in the hands of a skilled team, the patient has a good chance of survival. The real difficulty comes later, in the next few weeks or the next few months; for, if the blood is not properly controlled, clots form and lead to strokes and death—or, as in my wife's case, the blood thins out too much and produces fatal hemorrhaging. Yet the record shows that many hospitals and doctors take an unjustifiably casual attitude toward the whole postoperative blood problem.

Coumadin is a derivative of warfarin, a substance that is used to kill rats. In therapeutic usage, Coumadin is valuable to thin out the blood for a variety of ailments: to keep new clots from forming in the bloodstreams of heart-attack or stroke victims; to help dissolve clots in phlebitis; to prevent clots from forming after heart surgery. Necessary and valuable though it is in such cases, Coumadin is one of the most volatile and tricky drugs, one of the hardest to control. It can take off on a blood-thinning rampage under the slightest stimulus, propelled on its potentially lethal course by changes in exercise or diet or other medications.

Much too late, after Julia's death, I was given a vivid example of just how suddenly Coumadin can run amuck. This was an episode that, except for a seemingly malign fate, I might well have learned about years before; that I didn't hear of it until too late almost seemed to indicate that my wife's death, as she sensed, was foreordained.

Robert H. Prall has been one of my closest friends for most of my adult life. As young men, we worked together at the Jersey shore and later for years on the staff of the now-defunct *New York World-Telegram and Sun.* Bob and his wife, Jane, and Julia and I had been friends since our earliest days of marriage. For years Bob has suffered from phlebitis, and in the 1950s an especially bad flare-up landed him in New York Hospital under the care of Dr. Irving Sherwood Wright, internationally famous blood expert and chairman of the International Commission on Blood Clotting Factors from 1954 to 1963. When Bob was released from the hospital, he was placed on Coumadin; but, since he never talked very much about his ailment or his medication, I had been unaware of it.

Only after Julia died did I learn from Bob and Jane how emphatic Dr. Wright had been in insisting on a weekly blood count. "If his office didn't get a report from the lab right on time," Jane says, "they would phone our home here in New Jersey to make certain Bob had had his blood tested on schedule. They bothered us so much I got angry with them once."

The wisdom of such precautions was demonstrated one summer while the Pralls were vacationing at Culver Lake in northwestern New Jersey. Bob had been out in his boat waterskiing and swimming most of the day, and the combination of sunshine and extra activity triggered the Coumadin in his system. The whites of his eyes became fiery red, and he began to urinate blood. A panicked call to New York Hospital brought a prescription for an antidote to thicken the blood. There was great worry at first that Bob might go blind from the bursting of blood vessels in his eyes, but fortunately the antidote worked in time and this did not happen.

Warnings against just such scary Coumadin reactions abound in medical literature. Coumadin is not a new drug, and its dangers have long been recognized. In the circumstances, since the medical profession seems so frequently to ignore Coumadin's hazards, one is compelled to wonder about how it reacts with the spate of new and potent medications whose side effects have not been so well explored. (Dr. Sidney M. Wolfe, director of Ralph Nader's Health Research Group, reported in early February, 1975, that a small number of studies has shown that 30,000 persons a year die from adverse drug reactions. According to some authorities, Wolfe said, three-quarters of these drugs never should have been prescribed. Wolfe added that the available studies do not deal with drugs prescribed for outpatients or with the 15,000 diabetics taking an oral drug that has been found harmful and is medically justified in only a small percentage of cases.)

As far as Coumadin is concerned, the bible of the profession—the *Physicians' Desk Reference* (1972 edition)—admonishes doctors in this capitalized paragraph:

PERIODIC DETERMINATION OF PROTHROMBIN TIME IS ESSENTIAL. NUMEROUS FACTORS INCLUDING CHANGES IN DIET, ENVIRONMENT, PHYSICAL STATE AND MEDICATION MAY INFLUENCE RESPONSE OF THE PATIENT TO ANTICOAGULANTS. IT IS GENERALLY GOOD PRACTICE TO MONITOR THE PATIENT'S RESPONSE WITH ADDITIONAL PROTHROMBIN TIME DETERMINATIONS WHENEVER OTHER MEDICATIONS ARE INITIATED, DISCONTINUED OR TAKEN HAPHAZARDLY.

How often is "periodic"? The manual leaves no doubt. It states clearly that a "prothrombin time test may be made every 24 to 48 hours for the first week; once or twice weekly for the next 3 to 4 weeks; and once semimonthly or monthly for subsequent longterm treatment."

The adverse reactions are listed as "minor and major hemorrhage." Side effects other than hemorrhages are infrequent, the manual says. Among these it lists "hypersensitivity reactions" and "an extremely rare reaction consisting of hemorrhagic infarction and necrosis of the skin."

Those explicit instructions make much clear. Obviously, my wife's blood should have been checked not later than the Thursday of the week after she came home; to be on the safe side, it should have been checked twice by then. Indeed, I discovered later, much to my amazement, that this is just what had been done in 1964. Though Dr. Economos had insisted on the once-a-week check, I found in leafing through my old account book that Dr. Pond's Laboratory in Asbury Park had tested Julia, as the desk manual suggests, every three or four days. There were the dates staring at me: July 23, 27, and 30; August 3 and 6.

Another major shock came as I read that warning about the necessity of careful testing after any change of medication. Just one change had been made after Julia returned home, the substitution of Tylenol for Darvon. And I discovered that there is a serious, unsettled question about the effect of Tylenol given in conjunction with Coumadin.

It is well established that drugs containing aspirin must not be administered with blood-thinners like Coumadin because they increase the blood-thinning effect. There is some evidence of a similar interreaction when Tylenol is used, but there is considerable dispute about just how serious this is.

Eric W. Martin, in his book *Hazards of Medication,* writes: "Anticoagulant response is enhanced by acetaminophen [Tylenol] due to displacement of anticoagulants from protein bonding sites." This means that Tylenol and the anticoagulants apparently compete for the same bonding sites, and since the anticoagulant is bound to a lesser degree with the ingestion of Tylenol, its blood-thinning effect is enhanced. Just how significant this is, however, is disputed. Probably the most authoritative study was done by the University of Maryland School of Medicine in 1968. This showed that 650 milligrams of Tylenol, taken four times a day, prolonged the clotting time of persons taking Coumadin by 5.3 seconds. The study concluded that this prolongation was too slight to have clinical significance.

Whether there are individual exceptions to the broad conclusion is the problem. Each patient's physical and emotional makeup is different; each reacts differently to drugs like Coumadin; even the same person, at different times, under different stresses, reacts differently. The most logical explanation of what happened to my wife seems to be that the substitution of Tylenol, added to the emotional frenzy through which she was going as a result of her hallucinations, probably triggered the runaway effect of the Coumadin. And, of course, the clear warning in the *Physicians' Desk Reference* that extra care must be taken to check the blood when medication is changed was ignored.

Similarly ignored were some of the manual's other items of guidance and advice. There was the reference to "hypersensitivity"—I remembered Julia's complaint that last Friday night that her body felt sore all over. There was the emphasis on the major danger of hemorrhaging, and the unlikelihood of "necrosis of the skin." In the casual nonbriefing in New York Hospital, we had been told only about the symptoms that hardly needed to be brought to our attention. We were given no information about other symptoms that we were less likely to notice, and that were not dependent on injury.

What we should have been told has been spelled out clearly by Mrs. Ruth Mayer Shapiro, clinical research nurse in heparin therapy at Beth Israel Hospital in Boston. Writing in *American Nursing* (March, 1947), she says: "Patients and their families . . . should be taught to recognize these danger signs: darkened urine or frank hematuria; black, tarry stools; abdominal or flank pain; increased menstrual bleeding; joint pain or immobility; *head pain or change in neurological status* . . ." (italics added).

The lesson, whether the medical profession likes it or not, is that the patient's family simply *has* to know, especially when the patient is sent home so quickly. In my postmortem research, I came across one sentence in the volume published by the American College of Surgeons that, had we read it in time, could have saved Julia's life. Dr. Edwin W. Salzman, associate professor of surgery at Harvard, writing on the danger of blood-thinning drugs, emphasized that, if the platelet count goes awry, *"intracranial hemorrhage is a major hazard"* (italics added).

I have a vague recollection—something to which I could never swear because it occurred during the tensions of that confused time when days and nights were running together in a muddle—that Julia complained to me once about feeling pressure in her head. She didn't make any particularly big thing of it at that time, but she did later to Barbara.

On that Saturday afternoon on which Barbara relieved me so that I could get away for a couple of hours, Julia began to cry and complained of pressure in her head. Barbara, knowing as little as I did, ascribed this to her nervous state and tried to soothe her, patting her and saying comfortingly: "Oh, Mother, don't worry. It will go away. Everything will be all right."

Had we but known . . . But we had not been permitted to know.

20

ONE BASIC THEME REPEATS ITSELF ENDLESSLY IN THE medical experiences that have been related to me by others after Julia's death. It may be capsuled: Great Doctors be not so proud; be not so arrogant; be not so cocksure. You are only human. Stop playing God. For when fallible humans become convinced they cannot err, they invite catastrophe.

It is an attitude that showed itself clearly in the conduct of our own Great Doctor in Julia's death, that exhibited itself again in the experiences of Mrs. Marks's family in Virginia, that is repeated in case after case—in so many cases that I have not room for them all. The Great Doctor makes his diagnosis; satisfied of his own infallibility, the accuracy of his conclusions, he closes his mind to all else. He becomes at times casual; since he cannot err, he does not see, does not listen, does not consider other possibilities—not even when his patient is dying right before his eyes. Of all such cases that have come my way, none is more tragic than that of a forty-two-year-old New Jersey nurse and mother who placed her life in the hands of one of the great surgeons in one of New York City's great hospitals.

She was a country girl, born and raised on a farm some eighteen miles from Binghamton in south-central New York State. Her husband was an executive with one of the nation's larger social-service agencies. Since he asks for anonymity, I shall call him Henry and his wife Margaret.

Five feet six and a half inches tall, she was a slim, brown-haired, attractive woman. "She never weighed much more than one hundred twenty pounds even when she was pregnant," her husband says.

"She was a very quiet person, a very private person. I might rage and carry on about things, but she never would. She was an avid reader, always taking books out of the library, interested in the arts. We had a beautiful home, furnished in early American style, graced with many antiques that she'd collected."

In the early years of their marriage, they lived in the Pennsylvania countryside; but when the opportunity came for Henry to take a better-paying job close to New York City, they bought a home in one of the better residential towns in Bergen County in northern New Jersey. Margaret, as she later wrote, dreaded the move into the bustling metropolitan area; but her husband says, "She never showed me any of the fears she had about moving, and she adjusted quickly."

A registered nurse, she went to work part-time in a large nearby hospital, earning the extra money that helped support their new life-style and provide for the college education of their three growing sons. Life, it seemed, could hardly have been more beautiful; then the blow fell. Margaret herself (sometime in April, 1972) wrote the story in a diary that she kept. Her account was in the form of a letter to her Great Surgeon; and, with her husband's permission, I quote it here:

Dear Doctor G,

Thanks so much for my successful heart surgery. My internist here in the village says that it [my heart] is in great shape.

A mitral valve repair was done by your team last April, just about a year ago. You worked well in the heart muscle itself, but my dear famous doctor, whatever did you do while going into the thoracic cavity? You never could explain to me why I was left paralyzed from the seventh thoracic vertebra down.

It had never before happened to any of your patients—why did it have to be me? It is now a year minus one month later. I am writing this from my wheelchair. I am what is known as a paraplegic.

Thanks again.

P.S. I was a country girl at heart. The big city has and always will scare me to death.

A few years ago my brave husband accepted a job very close to New York City. He, myself and three sons moved to a lovely suburb a short distance from the city itself. . . . How quickly we settled down to fertilizing lawns, to backyard barbecues, cocktail parties and making sure the bathroom tissue matched the tile without fail!

I went back to work as an R.N. in the local hospital—loved the work and the money. . . . In the hospital where I was employed, it was a policy to have a physical examination yearly. . . . For about four years this was done and all reports were negative and I was passed as being in tip-top shape.

About the fifth year my chest X ray showed an enlarged heart—and the examining doctor picked up a mitral heart murmur. The next step was to be tested and tested and tested!!! . . . Sure enough, it turned out to be "mitral stenosis." This involved the mitral valve, and because of calcium deposits on the valve itself it did not open and close properly—thus causing a lack of oxygen and eventually insufficiency. Usually, it is the result of rheumatic fever or a strep infection of some nature.

[For two years, she was treated medically by a local internist, but then tests showed a buildup of fluid in the right lung. A heart catheterization followed, and the results indicated the necessity of open-heart surgery. The Great Surgeon and The Great Hospital were selected; she entered the hospital on April 19, 1971, with the operation scheduled for April 22.]

Being a nurse myself, I hated being on the other side of the thermometer. . . . My heart surgeon after about two days made his appearance. Recently he had been written up in a national magazine for his success in pulmonary bypasses. I wonder if I still have the article. His intelligence was fabulous and I envied his brains. Always, I will respect that most of the specialists were in the same category. So much intelligence, they could never answer your questions point blank. Always, they skirted around Robin Hood's barn.

The usual routine admission procedure—X rays, bloodwork, urine tests and so on. . . . All I needed was the courage to go through with it. I did muster it up—unfortunately! This was to be a closed commissurotomy—a mitral valve repair, the "appendectomy of heart surgery." [This "appendectomy" analogy was the very one The Great Surgeon used, according to Henry; he "assured us it was an easy operation."]

I was scheduled for the 22nd of April, but

at the last minute some man apparently decided that he should be done at that time—and my surgery was postponed until Friday the 23rd of April. Who he was and why he took precedence over me was never explained either to myself or my husband.

My simple operation turned out to be much more involved. It necessitated going into the heart muscle itself—removing calcium deposits from there as well as from the valve—putting me on the heart-lung machine. . . . All told the surgery lasted five hours.

[Henry takes up the story: The Great Surgeon came out of the operating room about two P.M. "Everything is A-OK," he said. The operation had gone beautifully; they were now closing, and Margaret would soon be brought into intensive care. Then The Great Surgeon said he couldn't wait; he had to leave at once. "I'm flying to Chicago for a conference," he said—and vanished into the skies headed west, to be gone for a week. Behind him was disaster. When Margaret came out of anesthesia in intensive care, she was paralyzed right down to her toes. As her husband wrote me, The Great Surgeon, of course, "was not there . . . and no one knew what to do or how to respond. All kinds of reasons were given and many specialists were called to the scene, to no avail."]

Meanwhile, back at the ranch, I was coming out of my brief sound sleep, I could hear my husband's voice—but with tubes of all descriptions coming from my throat, nose, etc., I wasn't able to answer. I had a pad and pencil, and I remember asking for ice—by writing on the pad —also [writing] that my legs were numb. I know now that everyone assumed I had a "hysterical" condition—probably because of the nervousness and tension and fear I had built up prior to the actual operation. I believe I was in intensive care for 5 days and then I was taken to a regular room. I have no idea how long I was in the other room, but I do know that I went back to I.C.U. for three more weeks.

I remember nothing—but I'm told that I conversed with my husband and children and friends very normally. I don't know—that part of my post-surgery is a complete blank. I have no idea how sick I was—or if I was that sick at all. My one lung had filled up because I was not able due to the paralysis to really cough up all the phlegm and drainage that I should have been able to do. I had four bronchoscopies done at the bedside without anesthesia to break up the matter and open the lung. I don't remember them at all. . . .

[Henry: "She couldn't get the mucus up out of her throat. There were times I had to pat her back and burp her like a baby to help her get it up."]

On the Saturday before Mother's Day I dreamed I was doing private duty at a nursing home on the next block from my home. I couldn't find the patient's room—so I called for the nurse who happened to be in I.C.U. She in turn called a young doctor over who had been on the surgical team. I questioned him about my whereabouts. He was kind, as a young inexperienced doctor can be. Explained to me that I was in a New York hospital. Had had my heart surgery weeks before. It was a success—*but* that I was paralyzed as a result of it. . . . When my husband came the following A.M., I was like the valley of tears. . . .

Shortly after that day [Mother's Day] I was again removed to a regular room, a very tiny private room on the 4th floor—2 windows—and from each there was a lovely view of tan brick. There was a bathroom that I would never be able to use—and a bedside table. That was it—$108 a day—for what?

I arrived at that room—was thrown into a bed. I had a Foley catheter—no control of my bowels—I laid in a mess for hours before someone finally realized there was a patient in the bed. I had a bed sore on my buttocks—very deep and the size of a silver dollar. I would have been ashamed to have one of my patients have something like it. I lived with it for three months.

Never have I been so exposed, so ashamed, so mortified. Some days it would be 2 P.M. before I ever got water for my bath. Coffee would be brought in at 7 A.M., put on a stand across the room. I couldn't reach it. I couldn't move. I would ask the aide to put it by my bed, but she would say that it wasn't her department. . . . Seems like a wild nightmare. Well, it was!!! Couldn't believe conditions would be so horrible in a leading hospital center.

From April 23 until May 29 I existed in this atmosphere. No one had time to bathe you, change the linen or get you up. Private duty nurses sat outside their patients' doors—sleeping —reading or chatting. Heaven only knows what their patients were doing—living or dying!!!

God bless my wonderful husband. To him I owe my life. Not that it means much now. His love, care and know-how is the only reason I am alive and sitting here.

My life has been ruined by a "simple operation." Not only mine, but my husband's and my three children's. They have suffered immeasurably. Somehow—in some way—they will be compensated for all they have been through and what they may have to go through. Never will I go back to the greatest hospitals with the greatest surgeons. My opinion of the medical profession is nil. Doctors are not gods—much as some people think they are. They are simply humans and they do err, unfortunately!!! . . .

Perhaps it is bitterness that leads me to jot down these little happenings. I am not sure. All I know is that a slip of the scalpel or an over-clamped artery has made this past year a very sad, unhappy one.

For weeks—even months—I cared nothing about seeing friends. I felt like a monster on exhibition.

To have been so healthy and a part of this world and to have it all taken away in a short few minutes of time.

Never once did the surgeon give us an outright explanation of what actually happened. Only he and his conscience really know!!!

There are so many things that happened in those six or seven weeks of my hospitalization that I have my doubts of ever allowing a member of my family to be subjected to surgery of any kind. At one point it was decided that I should have a myelogram—to check the spinal column for blockage, clot or tumor. My husband refused to sign a consent—because of my condition. During the night I signed it—even tho' I was not at all cognizant of my surroundings or even of what was going on. I am surprised I even knew what my name was—or that I could even write. I did sign it, tho'. The next A.M. when my husband arrived I had already gone up for the test. Ten minutes later I was wheeled back—I was in no condition to undergo the procedure. . . .

To pay back my family for all my inconvenience to them is my aim. They have been fantastic and great and patient thru the whole ordeal. We have been thrown into debt—had to build an addition on our present home, re-do the kitchen to suffice for a wheelchair. Our whole manner and mode of living has changed.

So thank you again, Dr. G. I know how famous and greatly known you are as a heart surgeon. I will never understand how you can operate on a patient, repair a heart so it beats and functions normally, and have the patient end up such as I.

Thanks again,

A most disillusioned patient

Henry tells the rest of the story.

After Margaret was discharged from The Great Hospital, she was admitted to a rehabilitation center in Bergen County. There she endured four months of therapy, trying to develop what muscles she had left, learning to manage her wheelchair and to pull herself from it into a bed or onto a bathroom seat. There she was fitted with braces that ran from her legs up to a belt just below her chest; there she was taught to use crutches so that, with the aid of her braces, she could partially balance herself and drag her helpless legs along behind her. Even so, she could totter along uncertainly only with the help of a physical therapist's guiding hand.

It cost $10,000 for the addition and alterations they made to their home. Special ramps were built so that Margaret could maneuver in her wheelchair; a special shower was designed for her, as well as a toilet, chairs, and a hospital bed with a trapeze so that she could pull herself up in it.

"She was humiliated by her condition," her husband told me. "She had always been a very active person. She had always done everything for the family and taken care

147

of everything. Now she was helpless and couldn't do anything for herself. She was praying to die, no question about that."

In his love for her, he refused to let her hide herself away from the world as a freak, her natural tendency; instead, he insisted on taking her out for dinner on Saturday nights. "She was so embarrassed by her condition that she didn't want to go," he said. "But I was determined to get her out, and I would get her dressed and take her. Our friends were wonderful to us and treated her just as they always had, but she was always embarrassed at the way she was."

In the summer of 1974, the family went to Avalon in southern New Jersey to spend their vacation by the sea as they had been doing for years. Henry and his three strong sons would place Margaret on the frame of a steel chaise-lounge contraption; each would lift a corner of it; and they would take her down to the beach and immerse her in the salt water.

They came back home early in September and had a weekend cookout for neighbors in their backyard. "She seemed in good spirits, had a couple of drinks, and seemed to enjoy herself," Henry said. "But the next morning she woke up coughing and gasping for breath."

Their doctor, hastily summoned, put her on digitalis. But medication now did no good. She died before the week was out. "The doctors said that her paralysis put an extra strain on her heart; it was just too much for the heart to handle," her husband said.

What had gone wrong in the operation? Why had The Great Surgeon operated when he was in such a rush to fly off to Chicago? Henry never got an answer to such questions. He found that "no one wanted to talk about this experience. The communications gap from beginning to end was evident. They had all the answers and knew all of the details, but told you nothing. 'The less said the better' was the position they took."

The only explanation he managed to drag out of the professionals was that his wife's tragedy had been caused by "an anomaly in her arterial system." He commented, "It's some fancy word to explain nothing."

Talking to me months after his wife's death, he reflected sadly on the way life had blown up in their faces just when they had reached that period in their marriage when they were looking forward to doing things they had not been able to do when their children were small. Their oldest son graduated in the spring of 1974 from Harvard, summa cum laude, Phi Beta Kappa. Their second son was a sophomore in college, and their third boy a sophomore in high school. "We had been looking forward to being able to travel, to go to Hawaii, something we had always wanted to do—and then this happened," he said.

Shattered, he gave up his well-paying New Jersey job, sold their beautiful suburban home, and moved back to the Pennsylvania countryside where they had been so happy in the early days of their marriage. "With only one boy left at home, I didn't need so large a house," he said in explanation, "and so I decided to move out here and try to rebuild some kind of a life."

21

HE WAS SITTING AT A LUNCH COUNTER HAVING AN early-morning cup of coffee when the new issue of *New York* magazine all but rose up from the nearby rack and hit him in the face. The cover bore this title above my name: "The Unnecessary Death of My Wife." And below in bold, red type: "THE OPERATION WAS A SUCCESS BUT THE PATIENT DIED."

He was a tall, thoughtful, capable man, and we had known each other long years ago when I was a young city editor and he a young reporter. After World War II, he had gone into public relations work, and recently he had been involved in fund-raising appeals for one of the larger and better New Jersey hospitals, one whose staff he admired and whose care of patients he felt was excellent. After he had recovered from his first shock and read my account of Julia's death, he wrote me:

> For the last two days I have been thinking of how best to tell you that, along with all your other friends, my wife and I express heartfelt sympathy to you and your family. But you should also know that I have never read an article in recent years that has so deeply disturbed me.

It disturbed me, of course, because I have known you over the years and wish that I had come to know Julia better than I did . . . because I am now recuperating from surgery and several times at home have felt helpless because I believed we did not have all the information . . . but mostly because I have worked for a hospital and know that cases such as Julia's are all too frequent.

Your key word was "fragmentation." We can take our car back to the dealer and say, "It isn't running right. Fix it," with some reasonable assurance that he will try at least to give us an explanation of what's wrong. Why can't we, then, have a health care system where we can take our body and say, "I don't feel good. Make me feel better"? [Why can't we] expect that the person or group responsible for us will be completely in charge of our case, even if it involves surgery or therapy at a distant medical center, and will follow the case all the way, attending to every detail of postoperative care and home recovery?

A major reason that we do not have such a common-sense, practical system—one so essential to life and survival—was indicated, perhaps, in the shocked reaction of another old-time professional friend. This friend, now employed by an organization that seeks to provide the medical profession with the latest technical information, wrote:

Strange thing is that I'm involved in post-graduate medical education. We organize symposia for doctors and have never had a failure. Almost never. We flopped totally, just once, when we tried to hold a symposium on Patient-

Physician Relationships. Doctors want to learn (if it's for free) about new drugs, new techniques or pre-paid health care plans, but they don't want to hear about the human side of their job —how to deal with the patient's medical and psychological needs; how to clue in the family; how to explain or give simple instructions. . . .

The tragedy of Julia and innumerable others can be traced to the flaws in the medical system disclosed in these comments by two concerned and perceptive workers inside the system. Americans spend some $80 billion a year for health care, and wind up with a system so fragmented with specialties, so disorganized, so incommunicative, that unnecessary deaths have been estimated by knowledgeable experts time and again to run into five figures annually. Isn't there a better way than this? Wouldn't it be possible to devise a system that might have saved Julia's life and the lives of thousands of others?

A solution that is slowly gaining acceptance in more concerned medical circles has been evolved in an unlikely place: the little college city of Burlington, Vermont. There Dr. Lawrence L. Weed, professor of medicine and public health at the University of Vermont, has originated and put into practice what he calls the Problem Oriented Medical Information System (PROMIS). It is a method designed to supplant the traditional "source-oriented" system with its overemphasis on one major problem or procedure. PROMIS emphasizes the necessity for a broad-based consideration of the whole patient, taking into account collateral problems—psychological, emotional, financial, social, demographic—that may retard and even prevent recovery. One of the system's major objectives is to close the information gap by giving each segment of the medical apparatus complete patient information, flagged with appropriate warnings.

Dr. Weed, who devised the system back in the 1960s, is one of those shakers and movers who come along all too infrequently in the stratified, highly conformist house of medicine. And like shakers and movers in any profession, he is often denigrated and fiercely opposed by practitioners of the old ways, who are resistant to change and hostile to new conceptions. This attitude exists with an almost vicious intensity among some doctors in the halls of his own hospital.

Tall, lanky, intense, Dr. Weed is a dynamo of a man, with a mind that races like the computers to which he has wedded his information system. Words spill from him in a torrent, chasing each other as if propelled by a brain too swift for the tongue. And they are vivid, well-measured words, rich in telling metaphor and comparison; illustration after illustration drives home the intellectual content. Now in his early fifties and almost bald, Dr. Weed sweeps with long-legged strides through his PROMIS laboratory and the halls of Mary Fletcher Hospital, always in furious motion—a man with an all-consuming mission.

In the last thirty-odd years, he has served in nine major medical centers (Johns Hopkins and Walter Reed among them) as well as in hospitals in smaller communities. It was while doing microbiology research at Yale that he began to question the premises of medical practice. "In the laboratory," he said, "we had a definite problem to deal with; we knew the problem, knew the goal, knew how to check it. Then I would go out into the hospital, making rounds, and the difference was striking. Spend five minutes with this patient, examine the chart, give an opinion—then find out later that the patient had multiple problems. I'd pick up and examine the charts. You'd find no complete list of problems, just random progress notes that were often of little value. So I thought: Why don't we make up a complete problem list in the first place?"

He had an offer to become director of medical education at Eastern Maine General Hospital in Bangor, and he went there, taking along with him Dr. Harold Cross, who had been at the top of his class in Yale Medical School. In Bangor, the two men began to experiment with a complete record system, listing each patient's problems by hand in a notebook. "He was very organized," Dr. Weed says, "and when we began to check in this manner, we found that the problems came through to us as never before. It may seem simple, but it isn't. When you find that a patient has five problems instead of one, and they begin to interact with each other, it isn't simple at all."

From Bangor, Dr. Weed went to Cleveland, Ohio, where from 1960 to 1969 he was director of outpatient and special services at the Metropolitan General Hospital. It was here that he began a collaboration with Jan R. Schultz, whom he describes as a computer genius. With Dr. Weed providing the medical knowledge and Schultz the electronic know-how, they began to devise a computerized record-keeping system, able to give an instantaneous feedback of the latest information concerning symptoms and their possible meanings, choices of medication, the interactions of drugs upon one another and other possibly dangerous side effects, and all other data that might be of help in a particular situation.

Computers cost a barrel of money, and financing is a major roadblock in the establishment of such a system. The cost in a large metropolitan center like Cleveland would be virtually prohibitive; and so Dr. Weed grabbed the chance to come to Vermont, where, in a smaller, more-controlled milieu, it would be more practical to perfect and test his method.

There are four essential steps in Dr. Weed's complete-care program. The first involves the compilation of what he calls "a complete data base." In some respects this resembles the procedure followed in practically all hospitals when a case history is taken of each new patient. Such records customarily focus, however, on the obvious physical ailments: what kind, when, what treatment, the present problem. Dr. Weed's data base is much broader. He includes in it everything that may affect the recovery and life of a patient, any psychological, social, financial, or demographic problems. In one of his medical papers, he illustrated the method. If a patient is upset and crying, emotionally overwrought (I thought of my wife, who had "her little crying spell every morning"), attention has to be paid to it. All right, he instructs each of his students, granted you're not a psychiatrist, jot down on your problem list "cries easily"—and then seek the professional help needed to deal with the matter.

In a book that he has written for local publication in Vermont, *Your Health Care and How to Manage It*, Dr. Weed culls from his long experience specific examples of the disasters that occur through the failure to work up a complete problem list. It cannot be emphasized too strongly that the cases he cites occurred in major hospital centers, for the standard apologia for American medicine as practiced today runs like this: It is true that mistakes are sometimes made, that a surgeon has been known to amputate the wrong leg, but such things happen only in poorly run institutions; if you have board-qualified physicians and a top-grade hospital, don't worry —it won't happen to you. Our own experience, plus the tragic tales of many of my correspondents, gives the lie to that comfortable rationalization. And so do the incidents cited by Dr. Weed.

His use of specific cases to illustrate his point and convey his message has driven some segments of the secretive medical profession up the wall. "What is this doing to confidentiality?" they ask in righteous horror. To which Dr. Weed retorts: "Wrong question. The right question is 'What is confidentiality doing to *you*?' I opt for communication over secrecy."

Much of organized medicine objects that Dr. Weed's complete-problem approach wastes time and is too costly; but Dr. Cross, who still uses PROMIS in Bangor, argues that the collaboration of nurses, patients, and other paramedical personnel actually *saves* physicians' time. Furthermore, he contends, full understanding of a patient's multiple problems leads to quicker and more satisfactory solutions, and in the end to *less* hospital usage. His records show that, in the last three years, hospital usage has declined at the rate of 20 percent a year. One of Dr. Weed's examples illustrates vividly the savings that can result if problems are identified before a lot of costly tests are made.

A middle-aged woman was brought into a major hospital complaining of chest pain, difficulty in swallowing, muscle weakness, and exhaustion. No complete "patient profile" was compiled before the hospital went ahead with expensive diagnostic work, all kinds of expensive laboratory tests, and X rays. These failed to track down the source of her trouble. Only after all this had been done was this discovery made: The woman rose between four and four-thirty every morning to help with the cows on the family farm; then she cooked breakfast for a large family; then she made up lunches for her children and saw them off to school; *then* she went to work at a day-long job, returning home in late afternoon to do the housework, get the evening meal, and help with the last of the farm chores. She never stopped working until between ten and ten-thirty at night, when she fell exhausted into bed. And this went on day after day. Dr.

Weed comments that it was "no wonder she had problems, but they were only symptoms of her basic problem, her killing schedule."

More important than cost is the great overriding issue: life itself. And the failure to compile a complete data base and then go on to the second step in Dr. Weed's program, the drafting of a problem list to deal with what the data base has revealed, can result in tragedy. Dr. Weed illustrates with this example:

> A superb specialist became totally preoccupied with an excellent piece of vascular surgery on a blood vessel in a patient's leg, and indeed did relieve the patient's current symptom. He kept no complete problem list, and a nodule detected on the prostate on an admission physical examination was never stated as a problem and no plan was formulated. Two years later the patient died of carcinoma of the prostate. There is no assurance that earlier detection would have prolonged his life—but it could have.

By contrast, Dr. Weed in one of his medical papers illustrated how the formulation of a problem list may succor a patient who otherwise would have suffered from a too-narrow surgical focus. A gynecologist had removed the uterus of a woman who had had a bleeding problem. The operation had been "a great success"; and, as one of the floor staff reported, "the GYN man said to send her home." However, the staff doctor was disturbed by problems that had showed up on Dr. Weed's collateral list. There was a peculiar U wave on the patient's cardiogram that he did not understand, and the patient also had hypertension. Well, Dr. Weed advised, the two problems may be related, but in any event you've got to find out what causes them. As a result, he later wrote: "They took four adrenal tumors from the left side of that patient. Her hypertension is cured, and her whole behavior and her whole life have been changed."

The third step in Dr. Weed's system follows logically from the first two. It is called "Initial Plans" and deals with what can be done to cope with the identified problems. In this step the staff suggests what diagnostic workup or management may be needed and what therapy, including drugs or procedures, can be used. And, perhaps most important of all, Dr. Weed strongly emphasizes the need for patient education—"The plan for educating the patient and his family about each problem." The dangers of Coumadin, for instance?

The fourth and final step in the system Dr. Weed has labeled "Progress Notes." It is designed to close the horrendous communications gap between the specialist, serving in a perhaps distant institution, and the local doctor into whose care the patient is being delivered. The transmitted information details each symptom, each problem, each step taken. Unlike the many reports which tend to emphasize the surgical problem and how well it was dealt with, Dr. Weed writes, "The emphasis here is on the unresolved problems. Problems which have been resolved are written up very briefly."

In his book Dr. Weed cites a case that, as he said in an interview with me, is "a perfect analogy" to my wife's. He writes:

A patient was referred to a hospital for the service of a highly trained thyroid specialist. Elegant diagnosis and expert therapy were instituted. The patient was sent out with no record and no detailed plan which would tell him and his physician what parameters to follow, how often to look and when to call. The country generalist who didn't know enough to work out the problem in the first place certainly didn't know enough to manage sophisticated therapy without any guidance, and the therapy got out of adjustment. It was detected too late [the patient died]. The specialist blamed the generalist whom he had failed to guide and who was giving him referrals on which his practice depended. The patient was the main loser in the whole encounter.

As can be seen, Dr. Weed's full problem-oriented medical information and guidance system shakes up the traditional, each-man-for-himself way of practicing medicine. "Doctors prefer to see only physical problems on the problem list; they are neater," Dr. Weed writes. He adds that patients also sometimes resent suggestions that their emotional and mental attitudes are causing some of their problems. And so "both go on dreaming that most of respectable medicine is like a broken arm or ruptured appendix—an isolated physical problem that can be fixed for a fee without knowing anything about the person. . . ."

Revolutionary as some of these concepts seem to many old-line practitioners, Dr. Weed's system delivers three other psychic shocks that are like earthquake tremors to the established order. It puts the computer, as many see it, in competition with human brains and skills; it sets up a standard by which performance can be monitored (since the problem list is there, what did the doctor do with it?), a truly horrifying concept in a profession in which a doctor's performance has been gauged exclusively by what he himself says; and it brings in the patient as a full and knowledgeable partner in the handling of his own problems.

One of the most frequent complaints in the medical profession is that use of the computer dehumanizes medicine and threatens to enthrone an electronic gadget over human skills, intuition, and genius. Many doctors also rebel at being presented with multiple problems, the kind of psychological and social issues with which they are not equipped to deal. The physician will get lost in the computer woods, they argue; he will be distracted by Dr. Weed's system, waste all kinds of time, and become less efficient in dealing with the physical ailment with which he is equipped to cope.

Dr. Weed argues that it is ridiculous in this age of splintered specialties and wildly proliferating medical knowledge to believe that any one man can handle all of a patient's problems. Often, many skills and much diverse knowledge are required. For that reason sound patient care inevitably involves a team effort, necessitating a thorough, well-coordinated guidance system. "The kind of compassion that wrings its hands and sympathizes we all need," Dr. Weed agrees. "And we can get it from mother, brother and the corner grocer. The kind that cures ills and relieves the pain, though, is compassion in its most practical and useful form."

He emphasizes that his computers store the latest medical knowledge and that they are not intended to substitute for human brains and skill, but on the contrary to act as an adjunct, an aid to busy practitioners. Their 20,000 displays and 200,000 choices of medication are designed to help the doctor, to remind him of things that in his busy practice may be too easily overlooked. No man, Dr. Weed argues, can keep accurately in his head all the details of care for thirty patients in a ward and hundreds in his office practice. He needs backstopping.

Added to the great number of patients is the explosion of medical knowledge in recent decades; combine the two and you have the makings of chaos. Dr. Weed blames the educational system for its overemphasis on memorizing everything in a world in which it is impossible for one human brain to retain everything that is to be memorized. One who has graduated from the system, who has been trained to believe that he must carry *everything* in his head, will reach a point, Dr. Weed believes, in which, not being quite sure, he will rely on an educated guess, the almost certain prescription for disaster. He cites this incident:

He had a young student doctor training under him in the hospital. "He hadn't been with us very long," Dr. Weed says, "when he was confronted with this very unusual, difficult case. He handled it perfectly, and I gave him a perfect score."

As Dr. Weed was walking down the hospital corridor after examining the record, a rival of the new student doctor said to him, "Dr. Weed, could I talk to you for a minute?"

"Certainly," Dr. Weed replied.

"You gave that fellow a perfect score," the jealous rival said, "but I don't think you know how he handled the case. I was there and saw it. He didn't know what the problem was. He had to look it up in a *book*."

"Listen, young man," Dr. Weed admonished, "I don't care where he got the information. The point is that he handled the case in the right way. Didn't he?"

There was no answer to this. Weed continued: "Furthermore, young man, I think you should take a hard look at yourself. I know that, if ten years from now my aged mother came in with a rare disease and that fellow didn't know what it was, he would look it up and find out. But, on the other hand, if she came to you, you would think that you had to have all the answers in your head, and you wouldn't be quite certain, and you'd make a guess. And when you begin guessing, the chances are nine out of ten that you're going to run into trouble."

The computer, as Dr. Weed sees it, should be considered a tool that enables the human brain to perform more efficiently. Analogies pour out of him in rapid-fire fashion. "The computer should be considered an extension of one's mind the way an automobile is an extension of one's muscles. Without computers, could we ever have gotten to the moon? Absolutely not. It would have taken 2,000 years to do the calculations. Each patient is five to ten problems. Who are we to say we don't need the record? It is like a surgeon trying to perform without a scalpel."

Even more than the idea of the computer sitting there like an electronic watchdog, the manner in which the watchdog is programmed drives some segments of the medical profession almost over the brink. For under Dr. Weed's computerized problem system, the doctor is no longer the sole judge of a case, able to make the case whatever he says it is. Nurses and interns—"less well-trained personnel," as the doctors put it—make their inputs into the computer record; and the original data base itself is usually assembled by a nurse and patient sitting side by side before a televisionlike console hooked into the computer system.

The cathode-ray tube of the console is touch-activated. A typewriter keyboard permits information to be typed and stored in the computer's memory bank. With nurse and patient collaborating, the nurse activates the system by touching one finger to the tube. Lists of questions begin to pop up. Nurse and patient together run through category after category, pinpointing all the patient's problems, not just the immediate physical symptoms that led to hospitalization but all related factors that affect health.

Donna Gane, the soft-spoken head nurse in the gynecology ward, explains that many doctors reacted strongly when they saw nurses and patients assembling the data base and problem record with which they were going to have to deal. The patients themselves were sometimes apprehensive at first, she says, but by the time the record was completed almost all felt relieved and reassured by its thoroughness. Many concluded that they had acquired for the first time a clear understanding of their problems. This, to Dr. Weed, is one of the most essential factors.

"The most important of all paramedical personnel has to be the patient himself," he declares. "It costs nothing, and it pays off in the long run. You simply can't bypass the patient.

"Every patient should have in his possession at all times a complete printed record of every health problem he has had almost from birth on—and its treatment. He should have this available to take with him wherever he goes, instead of having it stored away in bits and pieces in various doctors' and hospitals' files. The patient should have this record at his fingertips so that he can read it and review it at need.

"It is possible that once we have open communication, and the doctor and patient set goals together and work through the same record, the malpractice problem may diminish, and we may begin to gain some real insight into the overutilization of medical care."

It was a statement that struck me with special force; if we had had such a record, I would never have forgotten the ten-year-old briefing about Coumadin, and I would have known that our highly capable laboratory had insisted on playing it safe, checking Julia not once, but twice a week. I would have known that The Great Doctor's once-every-two-weeks schedule was all wrong and represented a needless gamble with a life that was very dear to me.

As Dr. Weed sees it, not only are patients like Julia Cook victims of the system, but so are the doctors themselves. "Most doctors are victims of a bad system along with their patients," he says. "Doctors who make mistakes carry a terrible burden. Don't think that they don't pay. What professional group, according to study after study, has the highest suicide rate? The doctors. What group has the highest drug rate? The doctors. Their load is enormous."

The evidence at the moment suggests, however, that most doctors—convinced, as is only natural, that the system in which they were educated is the only correct system—rebel at an entirely new concept like PROMIS. Even though variations of Dr. Weed's method are being tried out by physicians in more than twenty states, even though delegations of French and Canadian doctors have come to Vermont intrigued by PROMIS's possibilities, the doctors in the gynecology ward in Dr. Weed's own hospital rose in revolt in late 1974.

Donna Gane takes up the story. She explains that the gynecology service was completely computerized from operating room to ward. As soon as an operation was finished, the physician typed into the computer every detail: the patient's condition, any special problems, orders for treatment and medication.

"The doctors hated it, complaining it took up more of their time," she said. "Perhaps it did right at that moment, especially if a doctor wanted to get at the next case right away; but overall it couldn't have taken as much time as it takes to scribble a sketchy handwritten order right then and to follow it up, perhaps the next day, with a full report.

"From the nurse's standpoint, it was a fantastic system. We knew everything by reading the computer screen before the patient even left the operating room. If she was in shock, we could be prepared to handle it before she ever got back to the floor. We knew exactly what her condition was; we knew everything we were going to have to deal with. We could be prepared. It was *really* fantastic."

But the rebelling doctors became ever more bitter, ever more determined to get rid of the system. There were constant innuendos intended to express contempt for the computer and the nurses who wanted it. Donna Gane recalls this incident:

"I remember, when I came to work one morning, I greeted one of the doctors by saying, 'Good morning, doctor.' And he snapped at me, 'Did the computer tell you to say that?' "

Finally a vote was taken on the issue—whether to keep the computerized system or throw it out. The nursing staff voted 100 percent to keep it; the thirteen doctors in the gynecology service all voted to get rid of it. The result was that the computers were removed—"We decided to take them out instead of having the system slowly strangled to death," Donna Gane says—and the gynecology service went back to the old hand-scrawled order system.

According to Donna, the difference in efficiency is astounding. Doctors' hastily scribbled orders are sometimes in part illegible, and they are not nearly as complete as the information that used to be transmitted almost instantaneously by computer. Donna recalls how the nursing staff puzzled over one such indecipherable notation in which, they thought, the doctor had written that his patient was "reaching septicemia," meaning of course that she was in danger from septic poisoning. What his note really said was that she was "resolving septicemia," meaning she was getting better.

Before the doctors' victory over the computer,

Donna says, one of their principal complaints was that they couldn't make their proper contribution because it was too difficult for them to put information and orders into the computer record. "But since we've returned to the handwritten system," Donna explains, "there is little evidence of any input at all from them. An examination of the first fifteen discharges showed that about the only contribution they made was the order for discharge. One doctor had one progress note; another, two. But in case after case there was none."

What did the doctors say about this? "The story changed," Donna says with an ironic little smile. "They pointed out then that this is a teaching hospital, and the input should come from the medical students and house staff."

The internal rebellion has placed Dr. Weed's entire program at hazard. The development of his PROMIS laboratory and computerized hospital system had been financed by grants from the U.S. Department of Health, Education and Welfare in Washington. Hearing of the medical revolt, HEW became concerned about further financing, which had been projected at $1.6 million for the next two years.

The medical department of the hospital, Dr. Weed says, is anxious to take over the fully computerized system abandoned in gynecology, but action has been held up pending a resolution of the financial difficulty. Some foundations have also expressed an interest in the continued financing of PROMIS; but, as this book was written, help from such sources was still uncertain.

"It will be just a crime," Dr. Weed comments, "if we are cut back to the point where I have to disband this team. The computer personnel we have assembled over the years are irreplaceable; they are highly skilled people trained in the system, and once we lose them, it would be extremely difficult to put together another team like them."

With the uproar in Dr. Weed's own hospital casting doubt on his system, HEW field agents at first demanded the virtually impossible. They wanted positive statistics showing just how many lives Dr. Weed's program could save compared with conventional practice—something that couldn't be determined, given the variables of illness and treatment, without some broad long-range comparisons.

"I told them," Dr. Weed explains, using one of his ever-ready metaphors, "look, what you are saying is that before you give me the chisel, you want me to prove that I am Michelangelo. But how am I to prove I'm Michelangelo without the chisel?"

His logic evidently impressed HEW, for in the closing months of 1975 a new, top-level evaluation team was sent to Vermont. These experts gave Dr. Weed's computer team an A-plus rating, and HEW decided to grant $500,000 to the university hospital's Department of Medicine to finance further evaluations, with promise of additional contractual support.

With this vindication of his system, Dr. Weed has been seeking foundation aid for a conclusive test of PROMIS. "There is a 55-bed hospital out in Wyoming that is eager to install our system throughout, and in a small hospital like that the cost would not be prohibitive. For a grant of something like $2 million, you could demonstrate what can be accomplished when everything is tied into the system."

Thus, despite medical opposition in his own hospital, Dr. Weed and his team are still battling and still optimistic about the future of PROMIS, a method that common sense says holds so much potential for mankind.

22

WHEN MEDICAL ERROR TAKES A LIFE UNNECESSARILY, it shatters other lives as well. The survivors do not have the consolation of knowing that everything that could have been done was done; that death was inevitable, that it was the way it was meant to be. For them, the psychic scars are deep and devastating, and life often just a pretense of living.

A courageous widow in the Boston area tells of the death of her husband in one of the most prestigious hospitals in the entire Northeast. Though he had gone into the hospital for surgery, his was not an emergency case. Yet, when he developed a fever whose cause was never diagnosed, the surgeons decided to go ahead with the operation just two days later, on a Friday.

His widow wrote:

When he shot a high temperature on Saturday night, his first postoperative day, the resident refused to call his private physicians, and continued to refuse on Sunday, even when my husband was on the danger list. I had to call them myself because they were not to be disturbed over the weekend! Can you imagine the hospital not having enough ice-blankets, so that when one was ordered in a desperate attempt to cool his body, none was available! From the time I called his doctors at noon until he died at 6 P.M., there was such panic that they gave him massive doses of all kinds of antibiotics. For all I know, the antibiotics could have killed him. The post mortem merely said the cause of death was "uncontrolled temperature."

Her husband had been in the private pavilion of the hospital at a tab of $135 a day, with special nurses and "the most distinguished doctors." None of it had helped. "Can you imagine the doctors saying," the widow wrote, "that had they been called on Saturday night they might have done something to reverse the trend . . . ? Why on earth was I paying such enormous medical fees if not for their special competence, experience and expertise?"

She added, "None of that of course really matters because, as you well know by now, in one split second my life was shattered, never to be whole again." Though three years had passed since her husband's death, she had found that "It does not get easier—in a sense it grows worse. . . ." She explained:

In the early months, even though I knew it was real and I was shattered by it, I somehow lived in a fantasy world, as though after a while all would be the same again. I can't quite explain it . . . I cope, I live, I work—but the emptiness, the loneliness that no one else can fill for me—I yearn to be the center of his life, to have him worry about me, to love him, to share my thoughts with him without having to spell them out, to have him care how I look—to get pleasure in buying things for him, cooking the things he likes, and the myriad of other things that made our life together for 40 years and 3 weeks.

Perhaps I say these things to you because we don't know each other. I certainly don't talk about them to those around me. They could only feel badly for me—and could do nothing to help. I keep busy, doing interesting work—and amaze everyone with how well I "cope."

I can relate to that moving story, for Julia's unnecessary death caused similar traumas. For months afterward, one of my young grandchildren awoke in the night, every night, crying for his lost grandmother. As I write this, it is nearly a year after her death, and no day passes that I do not awake thinking of her, that I do not go over in my mind time and again, endlessly, all the mischances, all the bumbling—all those things that should never have been mishandled in any kind of competent medical system.

It is true that what I call "the great tidal wave" of uncontrollable grief has subsided a bit now. For months, when I walked the dog in the field, my mind, as if on some automatic pilot, would begin to think of her, of how marvelously well the operation had gone, of how she should have been restored to health and walking with me; and then that great tidal wave would surge up out of nowhere and come crashing down upon my head like some huge comber of the sea thundering on the sand. My face would begin to work and crumple, and I would glance around to see if anyone was looking, in fear of disgracing myself.

Little things—things that one would never suspect could be catalytic agents—would trigger that black tidal wave. For years, Julia had come to meet me at the railroad station when I was coming back from a day in New York. She would be parked at the end of the platform on the west side of the station and would drive slowly along to pick me up, the warm welcoming smile on her face, glad to see me again even though I had been gone for only a few hours. And so one day after her death, when I went into the city, I parked the car on the west side of the station; and when I came home, there it was sitting in its usual parking place, but empty. The sight overpowered me for a day; and even now, when I travel, I park the car elsewhere, out on the other side of the station on Main Street, so that I won't have to face it sitting there empty in the old familiar place when I return.

Holidays, of course, are the worst times. That first Christmas season was especially grim with its contrast between what had always been and what existed now. As Barbara said: "Dad, can you imagine what this Christmas would have been like? Mother would have been with us and feeling better than she had in years if the medical profession had only done its job. Why, it would have been heaven!" Instead, of course, it was emptiness and desolation.

I woke at four o'clock the morning after that first lonely Christmas, and the first thought that flashed through my mind was, How simple it would have been to save her.

That is the thought that harasses and pursues. How simple—how unnecessary. That is the true horror of it. It should not happen this way in a competent medical system; and if we are ever to prevent its happening again and again, changes will simply have to be made in the way medicine is practiced in this country. My *New York* article about Julia's death and this book have both stemmed from that conviction.

Doctors are going to have to stop playing God, and patients must refuse to let them play God. Patients must insist on knowing *everything* that affects their health and

treatment; they must realize that, no matter how prestigious the hospital or the doctor, stupid mistakes can and
will be made, and when they are, the patient and his
family must have the detailed knowledge to backstop the
professionals and prevent tragedy.

This is a concept that is anathema to the great ma-
jority of the medical profession. Doctors do not like to
have their imperial judgment questioned; they do not
take kindly to the idea of sharing their esoteric knowledge
with a mere layman, despite the fact that it is the layman's life, not theirs, that is at hazard. Yet stories can be
repeated almost endlessly of deaths like Julia Cook's that
have been caused in part by just such an obdurate failure
to communicate. And, by contrast, there are innumerable
stories of lives that have been saved because some knowledgeable friend or relative knew enough to halt the profession short of a fatal blunder. The experience of the
friend I met on the train the day I went to interview Dr.
Ebert, the experience of Mrs. Marks's family in Virginia
—these are merely a couple of isolated examples that illustrate the point.

The narrow fixation of the specialist, concentrating
exclusively on his one area of expertise, leads inevitably
to a kind of therapeutical blindness. The whole patient,
as Dr. Weed discovered, is hardly ever considered. Patients become numbered problems to be dealt with on
the surgical assembly line. They spend the number of
days in hospitals that records say should be sufficient for
their particular problems, and then, regardless of warning signs, they are cast off the conveyor belt to go home
and recover as best they can.

A woman who worked for several years in one of our
local hospitals, who has friends among the nurses, who
has seen it all, put it to me in these words:

"You have an operation; they have decided that this

particular procedure should require X number of days in the hospital; your incision is healing fine—and so off you go. They treat patients like so many robots; but the trouble is that patients aren't robots—they are *people*. And because they are people each one of them is different, with different problems of his own. But the doctors by and large ignore this; and that is why things like what happened to Julia take place all the time, and will go on taking place unless something is done about it."

In the year in which my wife died, the malpractice-suit crisis threatened the continued practice of medicine in many states. Temporary doctors' strikes took place in San Francisco and New York City, with physicians refusing to accept new patients or perform any but emergency operations. Such unprecedented protests stemmed from an astronomical rise in malpractice-insurance premiums demanded by insuring companies. General practitioners were faced with boosts from $1,500 a year to $3,500 or $4,000. Specialists, such as orthopedic, brain, and heart surgeons, were hit with prohibitive demands for premiums ranging up to $45,000 and $50,000 a year.

The explosive issue pitted the medical and legal professions against each other in a rare confrontation. Irate doctors charged that ambulance-chasing lawyers, deprived of a major source of income through the passage of no-fault auto insurance laws, had sought to compensate by drumming up malpractice cases. One study showed that in the tricounty Detroit area in Michigan, malpractice suits tripled in the years from 1970 through 1974 after no-fault went into effect. The medical profession denounced the legal practice of taking such cases on a contingency basis—that is, without any fee as a down payment, the lawyer gambling on getting an award and taking anywhere from one-third to one-half of it for his services.

The legal profession's response seemed to have considerable logic behind it. Malpractice suits traditionally have been the most difficult to try. They involve complex scientific and medical issues, and it has been extremely difficult until quite recently to get one doctor to testify against another; to obtain the kind of expert testimony essential in establishing the basis for a malpractice suit. Lawyers emphasize, therefore, that they risk their time and effort only on cases that they consider valid; they insist that they reject many more clients than they accept.

The malpractice-insurance crisis was precipitated in several states by the demands of Argonaut Insurance Company, a subsidiary in the Teledyne conglomerate complex. Argonaut shocked the medical profession by demanding premiums for 1975 that were two or three times as costly as those in effect; indeed, in New Jersey, it asked for a 410 percent increase.

When these demands were rejected, Argonaut announced that it would stop writing malpractice insurance. Chaos resulted. In the investigations that followed, several suspect elements in the Argonaut case came to light. It was disclosed that the insurance company had lost heavily in the stock-market collapse of 1973–1974; its losses stemmed not alone from malpractice awards. The company's new president acknowledged to a congressional committee that Argonaut had collected $35 million in malpractice-insurance premiums in 1974—and had paid out only $24,000 in claims. He added, however, that actuaries had estimated that the company would need a $69 million reserve to meet eventual claims on current insurance. It was a flat statement; there was no basis on which to judge the validity of such an estimate.

With many doctors insisting they would give up practice unless they obtained protection at a reasonable price, several states passed new legislation. Wisconsin and Michigan acted to restrict the size of legal fees in malpractice cases. Indiana passed a law the medical profession welcomed. It provided that a malpractice suit must be started within two years from the date of the alleged offense; it limited a doctor's responsibility to $100,000 and the total award possible in any given case to $500,000. It also set up a panel to review malpractice claims. Some legal authorities were doubtful about the constitutionality of a rigid limit on awards, but the medical profession cheered, hoping the Indiana act would set a precedent.

Other states, like New York, passed legislation to tide the medical profession over the immediate crisis, and the American Medical Association in its 145th annual convention in Atlantic City in June, 1975, mapped out a program to help state medical societies set up their own malpractice-insurance companies. In New York an expert testified that new medical insurance under this kind of setup would require only a 10 percent hike in existing rates instead of the 300 percent Argonaut had been demanding.

Thus the storm was weathered temporarily, but the basic issue remained. At the core of it, little recognized in all the angry verbiage, were the vital questions: Just how good is American medicine? Just how many malpractice suits are really justified?

The medical profession as a whole seemed unwilling to face those questions, to take a hard look at itself. It denounced the legal profession. It denounced greedy patients and deluded juries that sometimes returned verdicts in the million-dollar range. It pleaded for ironclad protection, for laws that would make it extremely difficult, if not sometimes impossible, for patients to sue. But there was virtually no willingness to face the fact that the profession itself might be somehow at fault and must bear a major share of the responsibility for its own present trials.

After my wife died, many friends and acquaintances urged me in almost these words: "Sue the bastards." I did not want to do this for two reasons: like many of my correspondents, I was revolted at the idea of taking blood money for the life of my wife; and I was convinced that a malpractice suit, however successful, would not help others. Such suits customarily drag along in the courts for four or five years; most of them, if they are legitimate, are settled out of court, with the whole business hushed up and the millions of patients out there none the wiser.

It seemed to me that, as a writer, I had the opportunity—and, indeed, the obligation—to try to tell my wife's story as a warning to others; to try to save, if possible, at least a few lives that otherwise might have been lost. That, to me, represented the only possible compensation for Julia's unnecessary sacrifice of life.

Publication of the article I wrote for *New York* in mid-November, 1974, did have some of the impact for which I had hoped. Julia's story touched the nerves of a vast and unseen audience, and brought me a flood of letters, detailing similar tragic experiences. The reaction to the article, according to Byron Dobell, my editor at *New York*, divided almost exactly into two hostile camps: the lay public, which was overwhelmingly supportive; and the medical profession, which was almost unanimously (in public anyway) offended.

Privately, some doctors let it be known that they understood and approved (but I mustn't quote them to their colleagues), and there were some signs that the profession was not entirely impervious to change. After Julia's death The Great Doctor no longer strode the corridors of his hospital so arrogantly. According to reports from hospital personnel, he went slinking around the corridors in embarrassment, fully aware that the whole hospital knew a life had been sacrificed through a stupid, incredible blunder—the failure to take a routine blood test. He stopped attending meetings of the county heart association's board of directors, and word filtered back to me through mutual acquaintances that he was a devastated man, a report that reminded me of Dr. Weed's observation that the doctor in such cases pays heavily along with the patient and the patient's family. After the *New York* article appeared and circulated through the hospital, The Great Doctor's embarrassment became worse. One hospital worker remarked to my daughter: "Barbara, do you realize who he is? He's *head* of the whole department, and he wasn't in the hospital at all for two days this week. Then he came in today, stayed for an hour—and left."

Finally, on the day before Christmas, I received word that the hospital board had met and replaced The Great Doctor as chief of the Department of Medicine. The announcement was not made publicly until more than six weeks later, when a routine hospital handout, published in the local press, disclosed the selection of a new chief without any mention of the man he was replacing.

In preparing this book, I was anxious to find out whether New York Hospital had made any changes in the faulty Coumadin briefing that had contributed to my wife's death; and on the remote chance that Dr. Ebert might be willing to talk to me again, I phoned his office. A secretary told me, "Dr. Ebert is no longer with us."

"Where is he?" I asked.

"The University of California," she replied.

It took me a moment to recover from my surprise, then I asked, "When did all this happen?"

"In December," she said. "Well, you better say January; he began January 1 out there."

In late March, 1975, I contacted a well-placed source

at New York–Cornell. He said that Dr. William A. Gay, Dr. Ebert's close associate and "a very conscientious man," had been named temporary head of the Department of Surgery "until we can find a new permanent chairman for the department." What had prompted Dr. Ebert's departure? I asked. He chuckled. "I guess he just wanted to live in San Francisco," he said. And so, when Dr. Ebert was offered the chairmanship of the Department of Surgery at the University of California, he took it.

Since my source did not know whether the hospital had improved its Coumadin briefing, I telephoned Dr. Gay's office. He was in the operating room, and I explained to his secretary, who recalled the *New York* article quite clearly, what I wanted. Two days later, when I had not heard from Dr. Gay, I called back, and the secretary told me, "Dr. Gay says he does not want to discuss anything with you."

I explained emphatically—and, indeed, went over the same ground two or three times—that I was writing this book; that I had called to give the hospital an opportunity to say whatever it might wish; that I did not necessarily want to quote Dr. Gay, but that I was convinced the meaningless Coumadin briefing had contributed to my wife's death, and so wanted to know whether the hospital had been motivated to upgrade this procedure. The secretary said she would explain all this to Dr. Gay, but if I didn't hear from him, I was to understand that he would not talk with me. I never heard.

The medical reaction, then, can be described as mixed, if not positively hostile. In our own suburban county, there were at least some indications of responsible concern, and an ability and willingness to change. On the larger scene, the principal reaction seemed to be resentment.

This, I am convinced, is not the kind of response that will improve anything; it will not save lives; it will not eliminate the fundamental basis of a great number of malpractice suits. With Dr. Weed, I "opt for communication." And for some fundamental changes in the way the system works.

If what I have written can in some way contribute to a better understanding by patients of the problems they face, if it can promote some movement toward change and communication by what is now a largely closed and secretive professional hierarchy, then Julia's loss will not have been entirely in vain. That thought helps, but cannot really assuage. Those of us in the family will be harried for a long time, perhaps to some degree forever, by the ever-recurring thought: How simple it would have been to save her if we had known. Then there would have been no need for the grave in that hillside cemetery in Brielle in which we buried one of medicine's mistakes.

About the Author

Fred J. Cook has been one of the country's leading journalists for the past twenty-five years. He was with the *New York World-Telegram and Sun* from 1944 to 1959 and has since worked as a free lance. Several hundred magazine articles of his have appeared in such publications as *The Nation, The New York Times Sunday Magazine, Reader's Digest, American Heritage,* and *Saturday Review,* and he has published thirty-five books, including many for young readers. He has won three Page-One Awards from the Newspaper Guild of New York for excellence in reporting and magazine writing, and in 1960 he was honored by the Sidney Hillman Foundation for writing the best magazine article of the year. A Phi Beta Kappa graduate from Rutgers University, he has lived most of his life on the New Jersey shore.